# PRAISE FOR
# *SIDE EFFECTS MAY INCLUDE EVERYTHING*

"Real strength isn't just physical; it's the ability to keep going when your own body is working against you. I've spent my life pushing through pressure onstage, but what Marisa writes about is a completely different kind of fight. Watching my niece grow up with autoimmune challenges gave me a glimpse into that world, but Marisa lives it, and turns it into something powerful. Her important book is a testament to her strength, her resilience, and her ability to raise awareness and help others find purpose and hope."

**—Davey Oberlin, producer/artist for All The Damn Vampires and Korn; @daveyoberlin**

"This heartfelt, candid, and often funny survival guide answers the questions we're afraid to ask about living with chronic illness. Marisa captures the messy realities of navigating relationships, work, and the medical world with honesty, humor, and heart."

**—Beverly Goodell, Executive Director of The Lupus Foundation of New England**

# SIDE EFFECTS
# May Include Everything

## A GUIDE TO LIVING AND THRIVING WITH CHRONIC ILLNESS

MARISA ZEPPIERI

A portion of the proceeds goes to MAHA Action 501(c)4.



MAHA Books may be purchased in bulk at special discounts for sales promotion, corporate gifts, fund-raising, or educational purposes. Special editions can also be created to specifications. For details, contact the Special Sales Department, Skyhorse Publishing, 307 Fifth Avenue, 4th Floor, New York, NY 10016 or info@skyhorsepublishing.com.

MAHA Books is an imprint of Skyhorse Publishing, Inc.®, a Delaware corporation.

Visit our website at www.skyhorsepublishing.com.

Please follow our publisher Tony Lyons on Instagram @tonylyonsisuncertain.

10 9 8 7 6 5 4 3 2 1

Library of Congress Control Number: 2026937530

Cover design by Marisa Zeppieri and David Ter-Avanesyan
Cover image courtesy of the author

Print ISBN: 978-1-63144-095-3
Ebook ISBN: 978-1-63144-094-6

Printed in the United States of America

These words are dedicated to the God who sees—who knows every ache, every unanswered prayer, every quiet tear.

Through the trials of my flesh, He has offered guidance toward my healing journey here on Earth, and the unwavering assurance that true wholeness waits beyond it.

# CONTENTS

# CHAPTER 1

# THE INVITATION

Picture it: the two of us, sitting in a quaint café in Paris. I'm shamelessly devouring a gluten-free chocolate-filled croissant like it's my last meal on Earth while you, being the dignified creature you are, savor your favorite dessert, crumbs and all. There's laughter, a bit of powdered sugar on the table, and a shared moment of joy and connection—even though we're about to dive into a conversation that's anything but easy: How do you move forward when suddenly handed an unexpected diagnosis? How do you navigate the world as you know it, *if* your entire world has now changed. I don't have all the answers but I know this: If we can survive these challenging and sometimes uncomfortable conversations around chronic illness, we can survive just about anything.

By the time you find yourself at the end of this book, I want you to feel seen, heard, and lovingly guided by someone who is not only empathetic to your situation but has also walked this bumpy and bizarre road before. Trust me, I've been there. And by "there," I mean that jarring, disorienting moment when your life is flipped upside down by a diagnosis and suddenly, everything—from *should I just shave my head now* to *did I do something to cause this illness*—is up for existential reevaluation. Because even in the post-diagnosis spirals when we question everything—and there will be plenty—I need you to know this: You are not alone.

Here's the thing: I want to have the conversations with you that I so desperately needed over two decades ago when I was handed a life-altering diagnosis. Back then, I was woefully unprepared. There was no such thing as social media or even blogs full of information. In fact, there was only one book in the local library on the specific autoimmune disease I was diagnosed with and reading it was like trying to understand an Ikea manual. I gave up after page three. Sure, my doctors gave me the clinical rundown but no one prepared me for how illness could, and would, infiltrate every nook and cranny of my life. No one told me it would shape-shift every relationship I have, alter my career plans, interfere with intimacy, or challenge the faith I have in my own body. In myself.

On LupusChick, the online community I've built since that time, I've often compared chronic illness to water—how it somehow seeps into every crack, every crevice of life, subtle and unrelenting no matter how hard you try to prevent it from happening. You can jam your metaphorical finger into the dam but somehow water still seems to find a way in—and chronic illness really isn't much different. At first, you may trick yourself into believing you can compartmentalize it, box it up neatly with a bow between flare-ups or appointments. Swallow the pills and not give it a second thought. But that illusion is going to crumble really fast. And when that denial phase passes, you'll think, *Okay, I am living with (insert diagnosis), so now what?* And that's where I come in. Well, really where this book comes in. To show you how to curate a life of meaning, joy, and purpose even when challenged by illness.

Because the truth is, chronic illness isn't going to be a single chapter in your story. It's the plot twist that redefines the entire narrative that *is your life*. And its reach? Well, it's vast and it's uninvited and the side effects and fallout from a chronic illness can influence *everything*—from your love life, finances, fertility, and sex life to your diet, career, emotional well-being, the ability to care for loved ones, and perhaps, most painfully, your sense of self. All of this can seem daunting, because it is. So here is what I want you to hold on to from this moment forward: Thriving is not only possible, it's within your reach.

I am living proof.

Even right now, even with a diagnosis, you are still capable of living a life filled with purpose, joy, and dignity. Even on your hardest day, when your joints are aching and you can barely lift your head off the pillow. On the days when your entire being feels like it's being held together by a band-aid and some dry shampoo. Even though things can feel so uncertain when a diagnosis gets thrown into the mix, have faith in these words: joy, hope, purpose, healing, and so much more can still be present here, amidst illness.

You are the reason this book even exists. So, if you're holding it in your hands right now, chances are you're navigating one of the hardest seasons of your life. Maybe you're in the middle of that maddening, limbo-like pre-diagnosis period, where every symptom feels like a riddle no one can solve. You know something isn't right, you know down to the core of your soul that your body feels off, but no doctor has been able to name what ails you. Or perhaps you've just been handed a diagnosis and now you're staring at the words on your medical chart like they're a foreign language, wondering what they mean not only in *this very moment* but for your future. Or maybe it's been some time since your diagnosis but you realize ignoring it doesn't work and you are ready to start living again, better yet—*thriving*—despite it all. Whatever season you find yourself in, just know I am along for the ride.

I've sat in those sterile exam rooms—the ones where the only thing colder than the exam table is the air of uncertainty hanging over the situation. I know first-hand the endless cycle of appointments, tests, and waiting for answers, and I've walked out of those fifteen-minute doctor visits with more questions than answers, clutching a pamphlet of basic information that didn't provide much solace. If any of this sounds familiar, congratulations, you're in the right place.

There's no judgment here, no medical jargon to decipher, just real talk about the things doctors don't always have the time or lived experience to tell you during your fifteen-minute appointment. Let me be clear: This book isn't about bashing doctors. Some of my doctors have been nothing short of superheroes. Others, well, let's just say they weren't my cup of tea. To be honest, I probably wasn't theirs either. I'm spunky, curious, and question everything (good traits to have for my journalism career). But what I have found is that most doctors are trying their absolute best within the constraints of the deeply flawed, overburdened system they work in. And even at their best, the truth is they *cannot* prepare you for the day-to-day realities and challenges of living well with a chronic illness.

Textbook treatments plus protocols do not equal or compare to lived experience. Our challenged medical system can't teach you how to navigate the emotional rollercoaster, the career pivots, the relationship challenges, or the countless little adjustments you'll need to make to thrive. They can't tell you how to sit with uncertainty. Or how to manage your body when it feels like a battlefield, or what dating will be like when your meds make you bloat like a blowfish. None of this is taught in medical school. It only comes from experiencing it yourself and gaining insights from others who have walked this road before you. And that's me, right here.

Some days my Instagram can fool people; I look like I have it "all" together, but the reality is that many days I feel like I just rolled out of a dumpster and I am trying my very best. Over the years, I've stumbled, scraped, laughed, cried, and raged my way through illness. I've had to learn how to craft a new career, keep my marriage, dog, and family (and plants!) alive, all while recognizing I still have worth despite being "sick." I've had weeks where I was too fatigued to stand up, days when I needed a home nurse to shower me because I was so ill, and moments when I've cried or screamed in my car outside of the pharmacy because I couldn't afford my prescriptions.

I've had to figure out how to advocate for myself in medical settings, how to balance work and finance with unpredictable health, become a full-time caregiver to an elderly mother, and even just muster up the energy after a treatment day at the hospital to make dinner, all when I could barely roll over in bed. No one prepared me for dealing with the mental toll of a chronic illness or how it would affect my relationships with family and friends. And don't even get me started on dating, starting a family, or deciding when (or how) to tell my employer about my condition. I honestly didn't even know if I legally had to tell them. But since my diagnosis day, I've discovered tips and tricks that have made life easier, and I've also learned what doesn't work—at least for me. We don't magically know how to navigate all of these post-diagnosis life pivots just because we suddenly get a name for what is happening to our body. These are the kinds of things you will learn in time through trial and error and from surrounding yourself with others in the trenches, soaking up their knowledge.

As I've sat in the trenches now for more than two decades, here's the first thing I want you to know: It's okay if you feel overwhelmed right now. Seriously. I spent more days than I care to count staring up at the ceiling from bed, thinking, *How on earth am I supposed to do this?* Whether you're grappling with a new diagnosis or still searching for answers at this very moment, it's a lot to process—emotionally, physically, and even spiritually.

It's okay to grieve the life you thought you'd have.

It's okay to feel angry, scared, or even numb.

All of those emotions are valid and they are part of the journey. It's okay if you seesaw between emotions because the fact is, when you receive a diagnosis, a grieving process occurs. And no grieving process is linear. It's not a checklist you try to blow through as fast as possible. In time you may work through the denial and anger phases, and as you feel yourself growing into the acceptance phase of grief, you may get really pissed off again because a symptom kept you from an important event or a flare-up ruined your vacation. This is part of living with an illness, so don't beat yourself up if you still feel anger, sorrow, or loss in the weeks, months, or even years after a diagnosis. I still see-saw at times through different emotions so many decades later.

But here's what I've learned: We are so much stronger than we think.

Even if you don't feel that way right now, it's a fact. You've already made it this far and that's no small feat. Even though your body is struggling and has likely been struggling for some time, it is continuing to fight for you—so I am encouraging you to keep fighting for your body . . . *and for your life*!

I'm not just here to help you *survive*.

This book is about thriving. It's about finding ways to adapt and create a life that's fulfilling, meaningful, and full of joy—even if it looks nothing like you originally planned. It's about reclaiming your power and learning to advocate for yourself in every area of your life. And most importantly, it's about knowing you are not navigating this journey solo. There's a whole community out there that understands exactly what you're going through and is cheering you on from afar.

In the chapters ahead, prepare to cover a lot of ground. We'll talk about how to find concrete answers if you're still in the "What the hell is wrong with me?" phase. We'll dive into what comes after the diagnosis, from career changes to relationships, sex, and finances—all through the lens of chronic illness. And we'll tackle other big issues, such as mental health, self-advocacy, finding hope when everything feels uncertain, and even falling back in love with your body.

We are even going to tackle the random questions you might feel too embarrassed to ask, like:

"Why do I literally feel like I'm dying three days before my period?"

"Do I legally have to tell my boss I have a health issue?"

"How do I handle that one family member who thinks I'm faking it?"

"How do I tell my partner I'm too tired/in too much pain for sex?"

"Is it time for me to get myself a shower chair?" (Honestly, these gadgets will save you an enormous amount of energy, so the answer is *always* YES to the shower chair!)

"What in the world is a functional medicine practitioner and why should I consider one?

Yep, we're going *there*. Real life, all up in this book. Raw and unfiltered (you can thank my loud, no-filter, and oversharing-prone Italian family for this).

And finally—because nothing says bonding like a healthy dose of vulnerability—I've sprinkled bits of my healing journey throughout these pages where I share insights on how I've been able to heal in different ways emotionally, physically, and even spiritually. I'll also share what didn't work so well or what I felt stalled me in some areas of the healing process.

That being said, recognize that my path won't be your path: Healing isn't some magical, one-size-fits-all, straight-line journey. It's more like a game of pin-the-tail-on-the-donkey—lots of blindfolded trial and error until you stumble on what works for you. Just to be clear, I'm not promising that if you decide to try some of the options I did, you'll suddenly be cured of your diagnosis.

What I can tell you is this: While I still deal with challenging symptoms of lupus, I've seen an undeniable upward trend in my health, strength, and joy over the past twenty years. I've gone from barely surviving the day, not knowing how I am going to shower, wipe or feed myself, to actually thriving—to living a life that's not just about making it through the next twenty-four hours but about finding moments of purpose, laughter, joy and still achieving my dreams.

I know the comeback from a diagnosis is possible because I've seen it happen in my own life. I was the girl who was basically sent home from the hospital and told to get my affairs in order, to becoming the woman years later standing on the TED stage sharing with millions that the world needs to start looking at chronic and invisible illness through a different lens.

So, consider this book your unofficial guide, packed with hard-earned lessons and "Damn, I wish someone had told me this" moments. Grab your favorite drink (coffee, tea, or hell, a shot of whiskey—that's my personal fav), and let's have the kind of honest, empathetic, and sarcastic conversation that can get you through even the hardest days.

Because, let's face it: Healing is really freaking hard, but it's a heck of a lot easier with belly laughs, shared wisdom, and a new ride-or-die who actually understands this unscheduled plot twist you currently find yourself in.

I've got you, friend.

Marisa
XOXO

# CHAPTER 2

# THE MYSTERY YEARS

If you're reading this, there's a good chance you've felt it—that gnawing, unshakable sense that something in your body just isn't right. Maybe you've been dismissed with a pat on the shoulder and have heard the dreaded sentence, "Your labs look perfectly fine." Perhaps you have waited months to see a specialist, praying to God or the universe an answer would be granted only to be completely let down, unseen, or worse, gaslit. If this sounds familiar, welcome to what I like to call "The Mystery Years." It's a club none of us asked to join, but . . . here we are.

The chronic illness journey often begins long before a name is given to the pain we are experiencing. For me, The Mystery Years began at the age of eight and spanned a staggering fifteen years. No, that's not a typo, though I wish it were. I often wonder what my life could have been like if only someone had listened. Fifteen years of symptoms that flared and faded like a bad soap opera plotline (I still love you, Telemundo!). Fifteen years of being told I was "too young to be this sick" or that it was all in my head.

Newsflash: It wasn't. And so, year after year of my single mother being told, "She's just a delicate child; she has bad allergies, asthma, etc.," the two of us navigated a medical system that often felt like a maze with no way out. We were poor and without health insurance and often—at least that's how it felt to me—cast aside and treated like a nuisance when we would continue to return because I wasn't improving.

But here's the thing: While my journey to a diagnosis was long and lonely, it doesn't have to be that way for everyone. My symptoms started in the mid-eighties, so comparing that to where we are today, the playing field has leveled up a few notches. Thanks to advances in technology, better awareness, and a growing community of patient advocates, the road to answers doesn't have to be as excruciatingly slow as it once was. That said, the norm is several years before an accurate diagnosis is made (averaging four to five years for autoimmune diseases, and even longer for rare diseases).[1]

Why are we still waiting *years* for a definitive answer? Well, there are several factors at play. These include:

- The fact that many of these conditions mimic one another in terms of symptoms.
- Sometimes our symptoms aren't outwardly evident by the time we get to a doctor—they often wax and wane.
- Not having the money or insurance to see the right specialist and/or at the right time.
- And in too many cases, we are just flat-out not being taken seriously when we do go to a doctor or hospital.

So, how do you survive The Mystery Years? How do you keep pushing forward when you are physically and mentally spent and ready to throw in the towel? Most importantly, how do you advocate for yourself in a broken medical system that often requires you to be your own detective, lawyer, researcher, public speaker, and cheerleader simultaneously? That's what this chapter is all about.

## That Rocky Road to Diagnosis (I much prefer the ice cream)

Living in diagnostic limbo is like wandering through a dense fog. You know your body better than anyone else and you know when something is off. Yet, the lack of validation from our medical system can make you question everything. I knew something was off at that tender age of eight; I wasn't like my peers. I was pale and yellow-tinged most days, black rings under my eyes, covered in rashes, constantly battling a low-grade fever, and exhibiting clear signs of lupus, including sun sensitivity, body and joint pain, horrific fatigue, and mouth and scalp sores, and still this wasn't obvious? And let me tell you, the outwardly visible symptoms at that age did not exactly get me VIP admission into the "cool" crowd at school. I was often called "the leper" and "skeletor," if that tells you anything. Leper was quite unoriginal now that I think about it, but skeletor honestly had a unique ring to it. He-Man was hot Saturday morning material on TV during that time.

If you know anything about lupus, you know the symptoms I was experiencing; the classic symptoms that fall under the criteria rheumatologists use to diagnose the illness. And yet, during countless hospital visits and dozens upon dozens of doctor appointments where I pleaded for someone to "help me," I was never tested once for the disease. In fact, it was never even mentioned. Again, this was the mid-1980s, when we had nowhere near the technology or awareness of lupus that we do now, but doctors *knew* it existed. It's not like I was patient zero. In fact, cases go back to 400 BC. That's right. Hippocrates suffered from the specific symptoms of a concerning skin disease that is now believed to have been the cutaneous (skin specific) form of lupus.[2] So, it certainly wasn't an unknown illness to the medical community. There had been plenty of people diagnosed with it by the 1980s. My guess is, I was way too young for any of them *to think* autoimmune disease could be the actual problem. While it typically strikes in childbearing years, children are also diagnosed with lupus. My point is that someone should have taken me seriously and dug deeper . . . but who knows, then this book might not exist to help you.

I felt like a human question mark for years, bouncing from one specialist to another, clutching my ever-growing stack of medical records in my Care Bear Trapper Keeper. That's how we rolled back then. Each visit brought a spark of hope at first—and often, heartbreak as I walked out of another door with no answers.

The reality is that chronic illnesses, autoimmune diseases, and most recently, long-haul COVID coming into the mix, don't come with neon signs pointing to an immediate diagnosis. Instead, they offer a grab bag of symptoms that overlap with countless other conditions. Fatigue, joint pain, brain fog, rashes—these can all potentially be symptoms of lupus, Lyme disease, fibromyalgia, COVID, or even just a particularly high-stress season of life. Add in stomach issues, and you can start questioning if it might be IBS, IBD, Crohn's, colitis, or a variety of other diseases. This is why it's crucial to become your own best advocate to get others to listen. And this "advocacy" requires some responsibilities and effort on your part. But don't worry—I am going to teach you to be an expert advocate by the time you finish this book.

## The Elephant in the Room: The Heartbreak of Being Overlooked

Before we wrap up this chapter, I want to talk about something I know is absolutely heartbreaking during The Mystery Years. You might be feeling this right now as you endlessly hunt for answers—the weight of feeling invisible. I know how experiencing this can make you feel like you just don't want to go any further some days.

Let's not sugarcoat it: Being dismissed is soul-crushing. We are creatures who feel and crave connection, and we all want to be seen. Whether it is from a specialist you've just waited months to see or your best friend or your spouse, the mental and physical effects of feeling unseen are real; the frustration, self-doubt, and isolation can feel unbearable.

But here's the thing: You're not crazy, you're not exaggerating, these symptoms are not in "your head," and you're definitely not alone. You know your body best and if you know that you know something isn't right deep down, I believe you, even if your Aunt Karen doesn't. And we will get you to the other side of this.

So, what can you do for your physical and mental health during these Mystery Years and those moments where you feel like you are going in circles with no answers:

**Get Those Feelings Out:** Emotions must be reckoned with because if you bottle them up, guess what? They are going to express themselves one way or another, and the last thing you want or need are more symptoms. Write down those epic nope-fest feelings you're experiencing—physically, emotionally, and mentally. Putting your thoughts on paper can be a powerful way to process them. Sometimes my friends and I plan a girls' night, pour our rage and sorrow out via pen and paper, and then sit outside around a fire with some tea and burn them over a small firepit as a way of releasing the things that we are deeply struggling with. Some read them aloud before burning and there are many tears among the group, and others keep the words to themselves, letting it end on the page.

If you are more vocal and not a fan of fire, maybe belt it out in a song that has lyrics that speak to you in this moment, or talk about your experiences on video. You don't ever need to post it unless you want to, but sometimes just speaking things out and naming your frustrations can be so healing. If video isn't your jam, consider a creative outlet like verbalizing it through a poetry slam or pouring it out through painting on a canvas (my personal go-to).

**Therapy is a Beautiful Thing:** I am likely the most pro-therapy human you will ever meet. Why? Because we don't have all the answers and sometimes a neutral party with a different perspective can be life-giving, especially when you are dealing with illness. The Mystery Years can often last a solid season in someone's life and you shouldn't have to navigate these struggles alone. A mental health professional can provide coping strategies and a safe space to speak your truth. If in-person therapy isn't accessible, consider online or app-based therapy sessions.

Also, as I tell people in the LupusChick.com community all the time, if you live near a major university or college that has a graduate psychology department, these graduate students must complete a specific number of hours of counseling to graduate. It helps them finish their degree and also helps you with low-cost or no-cost therapy. This is an ideal option for those on a fixed income. Reach out to your local university to learn more.

**Lean on Your Support Network:** Reach out to people who "get it." Major sidenote here: sometimes these "people" *will not be* your partner or family members, which can be heartbreaking but is a reality. Find the people you are safe to speak openly with, even if it's a fellow patient you befriended at a support group, in a Reddit thread, or an IG comment section. Even if they don't fully understand your symptoms or situation or are dealing with a different illness, having emotional support can make a world of difference during these Mystery Years.

**Perform an Act of Kindness for Yourself:** Whether it's taking a walk, soaking in a warm bath, or binge-watching your favorite show, find small ways to care for yourself every day. The physical pain, the pressure to find answers, the frustration of not knowing what you are suffering from can eat away most of our time each day during The Mystery Years. So, what is something kind you can do for yourself that takes your mind off illness for a brief moment? Personally, I binged *Frasier* so many times during my bedridden years, I can still recite many episodes word-for-word. It made me laugh, and my goodness, did my soul desperately need laughter in that season.

I would also indulge in a nice bubble bath where I would self-soothe with circular massages on my chest while focusing on positive self-talk, verbalizing over and over again, "I am safe, I am going to find the answers, and I am going to continue to persevere and get to the bottom of what is happening in my body." I'll be honest, I one-thousand percent did not necessarily believe this pep-talk at the time and sometimes it was hard to even get the words out of my mouth, but I kept speaking it forth. I believe it saved me from spiraling into the darkness on numerous occasions.

**Cling to Your Small Wins:** Focus on something *you can* control. I think this is especially important in this season because when we feel like we don't even have control of our very own body . . . well, we basically feel like we have control over *nothing.*

For this example, I mean focusing specifically on a task or to-do list item that is within reach. Something that is small and achievable. This could be as simple as scheduling your next appointment or finding an easy to prepare healthy recipe online. It could be Instacarting your family's weekly grocery list because you simply cannot fathom walking for an hour in the grocery store or paying a bill online. It might be washing your hair or going through mail. These may seem so simple, but in pre-diagnosis time, these tasks often took up most of my very limited energy. During my worst seasons, health wise, "bath and hair wash day" was like a celebrated holiday; it took *all* of my energy, I needed a nurse to help me accomplish it and I would sleep for the remainder of the day, but I felt refreshed and accomplished afterward. Something like showering—so simple for people who are healthy—felt like an Iron Man competition to me, and you are damn-skippy I marked that "small win" down somewhere!

Find something you can accomplish that is in line with your current energy and abilities right now. Celebrate that small win and don't let the weight of the current situation take this wonderful accomplishment away from you.

Last but not least, remember that being dismissed doesn't define your value. You are worthy of care, respect, and answers. Write this down somewhere you can see it every day—like on the mirror in your bathroom.

And hey, it's also okay to ugly cry into a pint of ice cream sometimes, if you aren't allergic to dairy, of course.

What's not okay? Us giving up on ourselves.

Our bodies are fighting every day for us, and we need to continue to fight for them.

## Seeking Out the Silver Linings

There's a song I randomly heard years ago on Spotify that has stayed with me because of the lyrics. The gist of the song was about keeping your eyes on what is ahead of you and to let go of the worry of what happened behind you.

The lyrics grabbed me immediately because they reminded me of the verse in the Bible, Matthew 6:34, that says: Don't worry about tomorrow. It will take care of itself. You have enough to worry about today.[3]

Both the song message and this verse remind me regularly that there still can be a silver lining in the midst of chaos if we dare look for it. It also reminds me to stop reliving past events that hurt me—the things that didn't work out or the answers I didn't get from a doctor I had put my hope in—while also not getting too caught up in worrying about a future that hasn't happened yet.

While The Mystery Years are undeniably challenging, they also present a unique opportunity for each one of us to be intimately present. Hear me out—this season of life offers us the opportunity to develop resilience, self-advocacy skills, confidence, and seriously, a PhD-level understanding of our own bodies. I am not saying any of it will be easy, but because of the unique and ongoing challenges this time presents, it's very easy to focus on and continually default to the negative: what went wrong, what didn't happen, etc. In fact, our brains are naturally wired to do this.

But what if we make a mental note to hunt out the good that can also be found somewhere in each day? The butterfly you notice outside your window. An unexpected call from an old friend. Or a level 5 pain day instead of a level 10.

## What Can a Silver Lining Look Like for You?

Maybe you spoke up regarding an area of your health for the first time today. Perhaps this season of life brought on the necessity of learning how to become an expert researcher.

Did you learn a new skill or take up a hobby while bed-bound? For me, being forced to stay in a hospital bed for long periods of time often gave me chunks of time to write—in between needle pokes and alarms sounding, of course. I talk about this in my memoir, *Chronically Fabulous*. While I didn't know it during those "Mystery Years," that season of nonstop writing would eventually lead to a career in journalism and book writing after my diagnosis. Whether art, music, writing, or some other outlet has become your lifeline, embrace it and consider it your silver lining.

And, if you are one of the more vocal types out there, perhaps you have begun to share your experiences and daily life with others through videos on social media. That in itself literally deserves an award. To become vulnerable and let people into such a private and challenging time of your life in hopes that it resonates with another person who may be struggling, that my friend, is such a beautiful silver lining. You are a light bringer and you never know how your experiences will inspire someone else who is ready to throw in the towel.

Silver linings come in all shapes and sizes. They are around us when we allow space to acknowledge them. Just stop for a moment amidst the chaos of your situation and reflect on something you accomplished, an area you see growth in, a small win, or how you showed up for yourself. Don't weigh these as "big" or "small" but rather acknowledge all of them as victories. Focus on the good here, all amidst a really difficult season in your life. Seriously, take a moment for yourself and a bow, if you want.

In closing, I know The Mystery Years feel endless.

I promise you they are not.

Answers *will come*, and when they finally do, you'll be armed with the hope, knowledge, resilience, and self-advocacy skills we are about to build together—all foundational must-have pillars to living and thriving with a chronic illness.

# CHAPTER 3

# EXCUSE ME, I HAVE WHAT?!

It's the moment.

That moment.

Whew. Nothing—and I mean *nothing*—can prepare you for that moment when a doctor finally names the thing that's been tormenting you. When I heard the words "You have lupus," I swear I could've thrown confetti and done a full halftime show with pom-poms right there in the hospital hallway if I had the energy. After fifteen years of being dismissed, doubted, and straight-up gaslit, I wanted to stand on a rooftop and scream, "See? SEE?! I wasn't being dramatic! Something really was wrong!"

But here's the plot twist no one talks about. While the relief is real, so is the gut-punch that follows. Because right behind my exhale came this tidal wave of *Holy crap. What happens now?* The atmosphere in the room turned heavy. My future suddenly felt like a gigantic question mark. In that moment, I was caught between validation and devastation, hope and heartbreak, answers and a thousand new questions.

In my case, a rheumatologist cracked the code fast—granted, I was hospitalized and my entire symptom circus decided to perform all at once, which was a rare treat. But finally, I had a doctor who actually *listened* to me. She and an infectious disease colleague ran what felt like every test known to humankind. A few days later, the results started pouring in and soon enough, we had answers. For those doctors, the timeline seemed speedy. To me? I'd been waiting over half my life. Literally.

If you have been diagnosed with a chronic, rare, autoimmune condition, or long-haul COVID, I need to start here: I'm sorry. I'm sorry for the pain, the fear, and the confusion you have experienced. I'm sorry if you have been made to question yourself and your body and if you've ever felt dismissed or made to feel dramatic or invisible. You've battled pain and fear while trying to hold your life together—and that is exhausting on a soul-level.

That said, I need you to hear this next part clearly: You didn't deserve any of this. You didn't cause this illness, either. And, you aren't crazy, "making it up," a drama queen, or imagining it. This journey is brutally hard, and nobody would willingly choose this path. It drives me up the wall when people assume people with chronic illnesses are "faking it," because let's be real, folks, if I was going to invent a plotline, it would be filled with tropical vacations, yachts, and a permanent spa menu rather than pharmacy lines, awful telephone hold music, and endless bloodwork.

## Processing the Diagnosis: *Excuse me, I Have What?*

While I can't assume I know exactly what you felt like the moment the diagnosis was thrown at you, I imagine it felt quite overwhelming, lonely, and scary, with a side of, *is this actually happening?* The moment the words leave your doctor's mouth, it's as though the ground beneath you shifts. Your mind races with questions. You may have contemplated in the minutes, days, or weeks after, *What does this mean for my life? Can I handle this? Why me? What will happen to my kids, career, marriage, and so on.*

Simply put, your brain completely spirals.

First, there's the emotional rollercoaster. You might cry, laugh nervously, or feel numb. You may, like me, ignore it all and throw yourself into your work, your schooling, your family, or your pillow. You may experience a situational depression season that involves a lot of sleeping and shutting everything out. None of this is out of the norm of possibilities. *All of it is okay.* There is no right or wrong way to react to this massive life shift. You may notice a wide variety of emotions taking turns in the spotlight. Grief, anger, anxiety, and worry might creep up in the weeks, months, or even years after a diagnosis.

I wish I could hand you a detailed roadmap for this new path you suddenly find yourself on, but after two decades in the trenches, I realize this journey is anything but linear and it's different for everyone. The good news? You *will* build your own map—piece by messy piece—and I will help you do it. You'll discover the coping tools, mind-healing strategies, and survival techniques that work best for you and that you'll come back to again and again. Because you'll need them.

What do I mean by that exactly?

Well, living with any chronic condition often comes with a lot of ups and downs, like riding a rollercoaster. Sometimes things are quiet and you actually feel like you can breathe. And then suddenly, it feels like the bottom falls out from under you and everything disintegrates. In those moments, you may feel defeated; like you made so much progress and then went backward ten steps. This is common when dealing with a body in revolt.

In those early years after my diagnosis, moments like this happened constantly. My body was struggling to find balance, even with treatment after treatment. I remember one stretch though that actually felt . . . well, hopeful. I'd made it a whole two months without a single hideous plastic hospital wristband—an Olympic-level achievement in my world. And then—BAM. Out of nowhere, a vicious flare hit, complete with mini strokes and a blood clot and my life came screeching to a halt. Again.

Months later, when the storm finally started to settle, a physical therapist began coming to my house to help me relearn how to use my body. My mission? Graduate from wheelchair to walker to hopefully walking again without a mobility device. I was in my mid-twenties and my "big" goal of the day, assigned by PT, was this: walk unassisted for sixty seconds with my walker. One whole minute, folks.

I was furious. How was *this* my reality? How did I go from the girl who loved to swim and spend entire days wandering malls with friends, to someone whose Everest wasn't some glorious mountain but sixty shaky seconds of walking on her own? Every attempt left me trembling, sweating, cursing under my breath, and completely wiped out for the rest of the day. While I wasn't angry at my physical therapist, I was enraged at what the situation represented. The loss. The grief. The anxiety. The absurdity that this was my life now.

All I knew—deep in my bones—was that I did *not* want to hear the words lupus or chronic illness or see another medical professional ever again.

Looking back at that furious, anxious version of me in the early days post-diagnosis, I see two things clearly: I had no idea how essential it was to grieve my losses, and I had never even heard the phrase medical PTSD—let alone realized I was drowning in it. It seemed like no one was talking about trauma, gaslighting, or the emotional landmines that exist around just getting the diagnosis, so I had zero tools to cope. Eventually, the tough shell I built cracked wide open. Just driving toward the ER could send me into a full-blown panic attack, because my body remembered what my brain tried to outrun: Hospitals, for me, often meant fear and bad news.

As time passed, my anger didn't settle—it sharpened. I spent countless nights alone in hospital rooms, arguing with God about how unfair it all was. (The extended meltdown can be found in *Chronically Fabulous*, so I'll spare you the snot-soaked details.) But one of those nights, my mom read me the story of Job and something in me shifted. I found myself staring down the question no one prepares you for after a diagnosis: If you lose everything—your health, career, independence, mobility, finances, even some of your "people"—who are you then? And how do you move forward?

See, we aren't just processing a new diagnosis in this season; we are also mourning the life we seemingly lost in an instant. So much feels stripped from us literally overnight. For me, I felt like I was crawling out from a mountain of rubble, staring back and wondering how I could rebuild everything that was just taken away from me.

Meditating on that question felt crushingly heavy, and I knew I couldn't untangle it alone—even though I tried to white-knuckle it for a while. Eventually, I hauled myself to therapy (emotionally dragged is more accurate, though honestly my body wasn't far behind), and I need to say this to you as clearly and unapologetically as possible: There *will* be a season—maybe more than one—after your diagnosis when you need a therapist, counselor, clergyperson, or coach who actually understands chronic illness. Not forever. Not because you're weak. But because some chapters of life are simply too heavy to carry without backup.

Here's the other uncomfortable truth surrounding this: Your ride-or-die bestie, your partner (who may already be terrified of losing you due to the diagnosis), and your mom (who starts crying three words into a health-related convo) are not the people for this particular part of the journey—they have other roles, I promise! I'm talking about a neutral, trained professional with zero emotional agenda or bias. Someone who can sit with your rage, your grief, your "I don't know who I am anymore," and your "how the hell do I survive this?" without flinching, fixing, dismissing, or gaslighting you. A person who can hold space, equip you with tools, and help you stitch together a version of yourself you actually recognize again.

Needing to bring in an independent party into the dumpster-fire that was my current situation stabbed at my ego and felt foreign, sort of like when you start a new school for the first time—you feel completely out of place and nervous but also low-key curious at the same time. But once I fully allowed it into my life and allowed myself to be present in that room? It was a revelation. Therapy was a whole new ball game for me. That sacred space was the one place I could stop performing strength and wellness and just be my true self, messy, emotional, and unapologetically honest, without feeling the need to edit myself to make someone else comfortable.

Therapy helped me start sifting through the wreckage and naming the losses I had never felt I was given permission to grieve. The grief in turn taught me a lot about why I felt so angry. My therapist and I dug pretty deep into the stages of grief founded by psychiatrist Elisabeth Kübler-Ross.[1] Denial, anger, bargaining, depression, and acceptance—they were all just waiting for me after I was diagnosed.

I jumped into the denial part immediately and then the anger came. But what I learned in time is these stages aren't linear and people may experience them differently and out of order.

What I also learned in talking with this particular therapist—who I saw for several years—is that anger is a secondary emotion stemming from somewhere.

I wasn't so much angry as I was *heartbroken*.

And, there it was—staring me in my rash-stricken face.

Heartbreak.

I wrestled with that word for a really long time once we deciphered what was really eating at me.

Today—after talking with literally thousands of patients over the last twenty years—I can tell you this with absolute certainty: When you're chronically ill, heartbreak has a way of crashing in like a tidal wave.

The heartbreak of *what could have been*.

The heartbreak of questioning if you did something to cause this illness.

The heartbreak of what daily life looks like now, and what could the future possibly hold if the future is filled with sickness?

The heartbreak of dreams seeming to instantly fade.

The heartbreak of watching the body deteriorate.

The heartbreak of contemplating your mortality and if you will lose your life.

When all of these questions come crashing through the mind, it is almost too much for one person to bear.

After becoming ill, is it any wonder we feel heartbroken?

I share all of this with you because if you are not already working with a therapist, church counselor, or coach, I hope you will genuinely consider it. Giving yourself a place to process emotions, grieve the losses, and speak openly about your fears isn't indulgent—it's an act of profound self-love and self-preservation. There is something sacred about having a protected space where you can unravel, question, rage, laugh at the absurdity, weep, and wonder about the "what-ifs" without judgment. A place where the weight of everything you've been carrying both pre- and post-diagnosis doesn't have to be edited, minimized, or silenced for people who can't fully understand.

Navigating this new version of life after we receive a diagnosis is both a journey of grieving what was and reimagining what will be. While this journey can feel undeniably painful at times, it has a less paralyzing effect when you are equipped with the right tools and support early on the path. When you find the right person to speak to (and it may take a few tries), they can help you name what you've lost, honor what you're feeling, and begin to reshape your story with healthier coping mechanisms—ones that make room for acceptance, hope, and even meaning to return in surprising ways.

Hope might seem really far away right now. Most of us are never taught how to hold heartbreak and hope at the same time. I certainly wasn't. And while I wanted to be that person who tightly grasped onto hope, it seemed most days my mind would spiral about the heartbreak instead. It wasn't until therapy that the "both/and" approach to emotional experiences became a lifeline. This concept teaches us to acknowledge that we can feel two seemingly opposite truths exist at the exact same time. In chronic illness this may feel like:

You can be both terrified of the unknown *and* relieved to finally have answers.

You can both ugly-cry in your car about what the next year of your life might look like *and* still feel a flicker of gratitude that at least now you have a name for what you're fighting.

You can both feel shattered by the loss of your health *and* wildly determined to rebuild and get stronger.

You can both hate the circumstances this diagnosis has put you in *and* still have hope that something beautiful might still be ahead.

Hope is integral to our survival, and having a safe atmosphere in which you can discuss how hard this journey is can be one of the places where hope is resurrected: gently, steadily, and in a way that allows you to breathe again, even in the midst of uncertainty.

The neat thing about acknowledging the both/and perspective of life is that it frees us from having to choose a side. We don't have to *solely* live in devastation from a diagnosis or force ourselves to always put on a brave face even as we are struggling. We can feel more than one thing at a time, still holding on to hope without ignoring the hard.

In the years ahead, I assure you, hope will sneak up on you in the most unexpected places—not just on a therapy couch or on a Zoom coaching call. For me, it showed up in the form of forever friends, an unshakeable mom and grandparents who loved me fiercely, and a faith that kept flickering even when I wanted to blow the whole thing out.

Hope also arrived through music, through art, and through celebrating every tiny win like it was the freaking Super Bowl. I'm talking: a custom cake for graduating from wheelchair to walker. Screaming with joy as the walker got exiled to the garage. Driving again—alone. Taking my dog for a slow victory lap around the block. My first solo "trip"—fine, it was just to the grocery store, but I practically felt like

Dora the Explorer. Being able to work again when I was certain that chapter of my life was over. Saying yes to dates, girls' nights, road trips, and now—one of my favorite traditions—taking a full week off every year to travel with my besties for my birthday. Those moments were my oxygen in a world that often left me feeling like I was suffocating.

Because here's the truth: This chronic-illness-life can sometimes feel like it's breaking your heart in a thousand different ways. So, shouldn't we celebrate the heck out of every glimmer of hope that finds us? The more I worked through the hard emotions and embraced that messy both/and reality, the more I learned to actually notice, welcome, and hold onto those shimmering slivers when they appeared.

The both/and mindset was just one of the tools that kept me afloat. Another gamechanger for me in those early years was learning how to retrain my brain to stop doom-scrolling through my life. Because here's the annoying truth about the brain: It comes with a built-in negativity bias. The human brain is hard-wired to obsess over worst-case scenarios and replay every terrible moment like a broken record. Sure, that's useful for cavemen avoiding lions. Not so useful for chronically ill humans just trying to survive a regular Tuesday.

When you're living with a body that behaves like a surprise plot twist, that negativity bias can go into overdrive—causing us to ruminate on every past flare, panic over every "what if," spiral at what seems like the beginning of a new symptom, and convince us that the sky will, in fact, fall at our next appointment. But here's a hopeful twist: We can retrain it. Not by slapping on annoying toxic positivity stickers, but by intentionally teaching our brain to notice the good, too.

And listen, I know your plate is already overflowing with test results, new meds, and Googling symptoms you definitely should not be Googling at 2 a.m. But I'd be doing you dirty if I didn't share this tool, because it helps.

For me, it looked like this: At some point during my day, I forced my brain to hunt for small wins—*any* good moment—no matter how tiny and even insignificant it seemed. A peaceful morning. A blood draw that only took one poke. A laugh with a good friend. An amazing cup of chai tea. A restorative nap during a thunderstorm. My favorite snack. The energy to take a bubble bath. Whatever. I made myself sit with those "wins" long enough to let them register. Over time, that repetition literally created new neural pathways. Who says you can't teach an old dog new tricks?

When my brain tried spiraling about a new symptom or upcoming appointment, I eventually learned to interrupt it and ask questions like:

- Do I have any actual evidence that this disaster I'm imagining is about to happen?
- Am I in danger right this second?
- What are three good things that could come from my upcoming appointment?

Did it feel natural at first? Ha! Nope. It felt like mental CrossFit. But with practice, I got better at catching the spiral before it swallowed me whole. Gratitude helped, too—not the cheesy kind, but the grounding kind. I would remind myself: *Look how far you've come, Marisa. You're still breathing. You're still here. You keep fighting.*

On the days when I couldn't see any of the good, and there were many, I leaned on my people. None of this was magic. It was daily, intentional, gritty work. But slowly—one thought at a time—I learned to stand on the truth, not the fear.

If we are going to survive—and thrive—with chronic illness, we have to anchor ourselves to the truths that never shift.

Fact: We've already survived things that would have leveled others.

Fact: We kept showing up for ourselves, even when our bodies RSVP'd "nope."

Fact: We fought for answers in a medical circus that often tries to mute us.

Fact: Even now, we're choosing to seek healing, hope, and possibility (even reading this book counts as an act of self-love).

These truths are the ground beneath our feet. We stand on them—sure, shaky some days—but we stand, nonetheless.

I stress all of this because you will have your own journey and will find your own truths to stand on. I believe you will share your story years from now and it will be full of strategies and techniques you've acquired. Your journey will be a history of the wins you achieve, the hopes you recognized. Your journey will be filled with stretches of healing—and I am not talking about the "Poof, you're not sick anymore, healing" (though I am open to that), I am talking about the healing that happens when you do the work. How we heal our heartbreak about that "life that could have been," little pieces at a time. As we heal the emotional pain, it physiologically helps our physical pain (more on that later). Minute by minute, day by day, we have the power to slowly rebuild.

In time, we stretch out our hand to the next person, coming in behind us—spiraling in overwhelm, where we once stood. And we love on them. And in our collective voice we say: This is both really difficult *and* you can still build an incredible life despite it all.

We aren't cured, but we are building a beautiful life beyond this diagnosis.

Together.

## CHAPTER 4

# THE DOCTOR WILL SEE YOUR DATA NOW

It's no secret: Chronic illness means an absurd number of medical appointments—probably enough to fill ten lifetimes. As we attend one after another, we're expected to pour our hearts out, explain years of symptoms, ask all the right questions, and somehow get answers, plus do it *all* in the whopping fifteen to eighteen minutes we're handed on average. Wild, right?

If you've never heard the phrase "appointment strategy," don't feel bad; I didn't think about "appointment strategy" or really consider the dos and don'ts of it all until doctor visits basically became my entire social calendar. (Spoiler: 0/10, do not recommend.) But over time, I learned what actually works in those tiny windows of face-to-face care, and I'm sharing my best tips with you here.

So, whether you're still trapped in The Mystery Years or you finally have a name for what's happening in your body, these tools will help you advocate for yourself like a boss, be heard, and make every minute count. Because here's the truth: When we walk into a doctor's appointment unprepared, our often-defunct medical system can eat us alive. But when we show up with clarity, questions, data, and confidence, the entire energy shifts. I've witnessed it firsthand. Doctors listen differently. We make space for better care to occur. We actually leave with answers and/or a plan instead of frustration and feeling defeated.

The advice here isn't about learning how to be a "good patient"—it's about being armed with knowledge and intentional, tangible actions we can begin today to get what we deserve: competent, compassionate, *collaborative* care. We are going to dig into various types of patient-obtained medical data and how to actively instill it into your health journey. If you're asking, "Why is data so important?" think about it like this: If living with a chronic illness is like watching one very long, anxiety-inducing movie, condensed medical data is like watching the YouTube shorts version. It takes all of the fuzzy scenes of our medical journey and turns them into a coherent short story. So buckle up and think of this chapter as your cheat sheet for turning lived experience into clinical leverage—and for blossoming into the kind of patient who leaves appointments with answers, not a frustrated text to yourself at 4 a.m. about what you should have said.

## The Life-Giving Power of Your Voice + Data

I know, I know . . . those days, weeks, and literally sometimes months you are waiting to see a doctor or specialist can feel like you've been sucked into some kind of sloth-speed time warp, but there is something you can do during the waiting that can prove to be most helpful: track your data. You're probably thinking, *boring, Marisa*! But hear me out: Think of yourself as undercover—CIA-level agent status.

You're on a mission and every symptom note is a clue. The more precise your evidence, the faster a medical professional might be able to connect the dots. And no, "I've been tired" isn't enough of a clue to use in cases like ours. Doctors need actual data—they love data! The more you can provide them, the more likely you are giving them the clues they need to solve the problem.

Because we wait so long for the "blink-once-and-it's-over appointment," we need to use this time as intentionally as possible. Before we nerd out on the types of data to collect and the best ways to track this data, I want to first shift how you think about one crucial piece of the appointment: *How* you speak in that room can completely change your treatment. To prove my theory, let's play out two versions of the exact same conversation with a doctor—same symptoms, same person—except in one conversation she's quite vague, and in the other she's armed with data. For context, in this example the patient is experiencing early lupus symptoms but hasn't been diagnosed yet.

### *Conversation #1:*

**Doctor:** "Please tell me what has been bothering you lately."
**Patient:** "Well, I've been really tired and just not feeling like myself. I have no energy and just haven't had a lot of motivation for school and work, and I'm always hot and itchy. I sleep so much, too, which isn't like me. I had a weird spot on my tongue a few months ago and I just feel strange."

The above statement does showcase a patient self-reporting—they provide a subjective description of their health status—and while this is a great place to begin, the answer is somewhat vague. It does offer a starting point by mentioning fatigue and lack of energy, but then it travels in a variety of directions. Don't get me wrong, this is still a good starting point and can get the ball rolling in terms of treatment/diagnosis, but there is serious room for improvement in this example.

Now let's see another version of this conversation, one where the patient is speaking with more confidence as she is armed with Patient Generated Health Data or PGHD. This is data typically obtained from wearable devices, fitness trackers and health apps, as well as journaling and health diaries.

### *Conversation #2:*

**Doctor:** "Explain what has been bothering you lately."

**Patient:** "I've noticed a major change in how I feel over the past three months. According to my Apple watch/Fitbit, I am sleeping upwards of twelve to thirteen hours a day, five to six days per week, and I am still exhausted. For the past month, I no longer have the energy to complete everyday tasks such as cooking, grocery shopping, cleaning, showering and working. Also, according to my health tracking app, I've had a fever above 100 degrees ten out of the past twenty days, and I've noticed sores on my tongue. Through my personal journaling, I've noticed the fever and sores seem to occur shortly after I'm in the heat or sun. I have photos of the sores because I wasn't sure if they would still be present by the time this appointment occurred."

This response might seem overwhelming, but trust me, there is pure gold here. Let's break this version down and look at key points:

"I've noticed a major change in how I feel over the past three months."

Have you been feeling ill for three days, weeks, or three months? The time frame will be a key factor for the physician as he/she starts to consider all the pieces of the puzzle. In this conversation, the patient lays a foundation through providing a specific range of time since her health changed.

"According to my Apple watch/Fitbit, I am sleeping upwards of twelve to thirteen hours a day, five to six days per week, and I am still exhausted."

In the world of medicine, tired does not equal fatigue. Tiredness is considered a temporary state, typically due to stress, lack of sleep, or overexertion. Fatigue, on the other hand, is a more persistent lack of energy that is often severe and begins to interfere with your daily life (more on that in a moment). In the example above, the doctor understands the patient has electronically been tracking her sleep, she is sleeping much longer than the average person typically needs, and that even with adequate sleep, her energy levels have not improved.

"I do not have the energy any longer to complete everyday tasks such as cooking, grocery shopping, cleaning, showering and working."

The above sentence might not seem all that important, but I personally believe it is one of the most crucial in this entire conversation. Back when I was in nursing school, my professors drove home the phrase "Activities of Daily Living" (ADLs), an evaluation tool to determine function status and severity of illness or disability. ADLs are tasks such as taking care of one's personal hygiene, dressing, eating, cleaning, mobility, etc. The higher one's level of inability to perform these tasks, typically the higher the level of severity of illness or frailty. This sentence above gives the doctor a clear picture that symptoms have become severe enough to interfere with ADLs.

"Also, according to my health tracking app, I've reported a fever above 100 degrees ten out of the past twenty days, and I've noticed sores on my tongue. Through my personal journaling, I've noticed the fever and sores seem to occur shortly after I'm in the heat or sun."

Here, the patient combines self-reporting with app tracking data regarding specific symptoms. Did she have a fever *or* did she have a fever over 100 degrees for ten days? One of these answers provides much more data. Sores are also a specific symptom to mention, and by providing the area of the body where the sores erupted allows a physician to rule out certain diseases. Last, she mentions that through journaling (a topic we will explore shortly), she noticed a correlation that when exposed to the sun or heat, symptoms present shortly after.

"I have photos of the sores because I wasn't sure if they would still be present by the time this appointment occurred."

If there's one takeaway in this entire conversation, this would be the clincher for me. Anyone who has ever swum in the choppy seas of chronic illness knows this: Not every symptom you deal with during that waiting period to see your doctor will be visible or occurring the day you actually see the doctor. So, the veteran journalist in me is shouting the following sentence loudly: **Document everything through pictures and video whenever possible!**

So many doctors have told me over the years that my notes, exported tracking reports, and—perhaps most surprisingly—photos and videos were game-changers. Twice those visuals were practically lifesaving: They helped clinch diagnoses for chronic urticaria (hives that spread from my legs to my face) and for lupus vasculitis. The two conditions looked wildly different and evolved on different timelines, but the videos and photos captured the shifting patterns and color changes over days—evidence no doctor could argue with. Trust me: A short video or time-stamped photo series is Sherlock-level evidence that speaks louder than a thousand words.

## Health Trackers and Apps: Two Must-Have Tools in the Chronic Illness War Chest

In your conversations with doctors, self-reported information will vary and might include a variety of trackable data such as weight gain or loss, timestamps of glucose readings, O2 saturation information, blood pressure readings, heart rate, and more. Two ways to obtain as much information as possible are health tracking apps and devices, and daily journaling. Let's dig in:

First, let's talk about gadgets and apps. One of the easiest ways to start collecting meaningful medical data is with trackers and apps. There are countless symptom apps at our fingertips (think Folia Health—my personal favorite, Bearable, Flaredown, and mySymptoms) that let you log pain, fatigue, meds, and triggers like food. With even just a few minutes of research, you'll find each app tends to offer assistance with something specific like physical symptoms, food sensitivities, mental health and/or sleep. Choose the ones that align with your symptoms or conditions.

In addition to apps, we have a wide variety of wearables (Apple Watch, Fitbit, Garmin, Oura) that quietly collect steps, sleep, resting heart rate, heart rate variables, and sometimes $SpO_2$ or skin temperature. Round these out with medical-grade consumer devices that give you objective vitals: blood pressure cuffs, pulse oximeters, Dexcom CGMs for glucose levels, and even things like instant EKG tools that fit in your purse thanks to brands like KardiaMobile ECG (I never leave home without this product). A handy feature with many of these apps and tools is the ability to export reports or screenshots—either through an in-app dashboard or by exporting CSV/PDF files. These will come in handy later when speaking with your doctor or creating your "snapshot" for your upcoming appointment (more on that shortly).

What I would stress to you regarding any of the tools mentioned above is to pick tools that match your lifestyle and comfort level. If you aren't a fan of continuously wearing a tracking ring or watch, an app may be better suited for you. But if you do opt for a wearable and you are also someone who uses apps, be sure to check for interoperability—ensuring the app can speak directly to your Apple Watch/ Fitbit or Android/iPhone and can help you consolidate data.

Finally, here's a quick privacy PSA before you go into full-tech mode. Be sure to read the fine print when signing up and creating accounts. Many consumer apps aren't HIPAA-covered, meaning unless you specifically opt-out/turn off data-sharing, you are giving permission for the brand to share de-identified data with third parties for research or ads.

Pick the devices and apps that are tailored to your health needs, know your settings, and then let these tools work for you. Let them gather the details so your brain and body can rest. A little setup and learning curve in the beginning means more clarity later—and that clarity can change everything about how you and your medical team care for you.

## How Daily Journaling Literally Saved My Life (and Sanity)

When I was at my lowest point shortly after my diagnosis, someone who knew I loved to write encouraged me to begin journaling about my health, specifically advising me to take copious notes about everything that transpired daily. I had zero reasons to say no, and so many reasons to say yes to this exercise. First, I was basically bed bound, whether it was at home or in the hospital, and second, my symptoms were wildly out of control. I couldn't figure out if I was coming or going most days. So, armed with a dollar store notebook a few days later, I began what eventually became known as my Mind-Body Manifesto. Let me give you the three-minute spiel about what journaling blew the lid off of in my life.

It didn't take more than a few days of scribbling to realize that if I was going to do this with intention, I needed to keep track of everything. Every day I would have a TMI session with this spiral notebook and there was nothing I left out—and in time, it made all the difference. My journal knew what and when I ate, what stressors were happening in my life, if I had an emotional outburst that day from the weight of it all, how much I slept, new or recurring symptoms I was having, if I was having my period, new meds or supplements I tried, etc. To illustrate further, here is what a typical journal entry looked like for me on any given day:

At first glance, you might be thinking, Okay, Marisa, cute charts. But how did scribbling notes about your watermelon intake and sleep schedule actually change anything? Honestly? In the beginning, it didn't. Not right away. Those first few weeks felt like I was just journaling into the abyss. But I kept going. Every day, I showed up for myself and a body that was exhausted, confused, and fighting like hell.

And then—slowly—patterns started whispering. Then began nudging me. Soon enough, they were basically jumping off the page, screaming, "HELLO, THESE ARE YOUR TRIGGERS, MARISA!" My daily logs turned into undeniable clues: clues about what sparked my symptoms, what soothed them, and what foods/emotions/activities/meds and external triggers sent me into a full-blown flare. In time, I started noticing the same symptoms crashing the party again and again, so I flipped back through my notes to see what else was happening on those days.

MY NOTES

June 2, 2002

**Main Symptoms**
*A.M.fever 100.5*
*new mouth sore*
*extreme fatigue*
*rash over cheeks*
*leg pain*
*short of breath*

**Activity**
*Sat on porch for 15 min*
****Walked around block in afternoon (felt feverish afterward)*
*Slept 10 hours last night*
*Took 3 hour nap*
*Showered - exhausted after and winded*

**Stressors**
*Cried for a few minutes earlier today*

**Meds/Supplements**
*List of all meds I took that day, any vitamins, new pills or supplements I tried.*

**Medical Visits**
*No appts today*

**Menstrual Cycle**
*approximately 3 days before my next period*

**Food/Drink**
*Breakfast -hard boiled egg*
*24 oz water*
*blueberries*
*turkey sausage*

*Snack - watermelon*

*Lunch -hot green tea*
*grilled chicken sand*
*mayo, tomato, wheat bun*
*sweet potato*

*Dinner - 24 oz water*
*rice and beans*
*skirt steak*
*apple juice*
*2 choc chip cookies*

**asterisk any new foods you try and journal if you have any reaction*

Then I went deeper. I looked at the moments I felt wrecked emotionally—meltdowns after particularly hard days, grief-soaked tears at a funeral, and full-body stress responses. I recognized the deep correlation between my emotional and physical health—the data didn't lie. Tracking didn't cure me, but it *did* finally help me connect the health dots I couldn't see when the entire world around me felt like chaos.

If you spend a solid season journaling, patterns will start to reveal themselves. Some of them will be neon-sign-level obvious. For me, these glaring patterns included:

**My period, and how it almost took me out every month**. Ladies, I am not exaggerating; three days before my menstrual cycle, my symptoms would hit like a tsunami out of nowhere. And every single month, I swore it was time to plan my funeral. I would get horrible fevers, incapacitating fatigue, crazy heart palpitations and mouth sores like clockwork, and these symptoms wouldn't calm down until my cycle had started and I was a few days in. It would take a good week or so to recover, and soon enough the cycle would start all over again. Years after the diagnosis, I discovered through research that this is extremely common for women with autoimmune disease because of the hormone shifts.[1] Today, it is more often discussed and finally acknowledged, but alas, not one medical professional ever mentioned this to me when I was younger. If I mentioned it to them, it was often dismissed as "not having any correlation." Today, there is so much research available linking menstrual cycles and other hormone shifting medical scenarios like pregnancy to an uptick of chronic illness symptoms, and I'm grateful we are in a world where you can finally access information about this link without getting side-eyed.

**Sunlight and heat: my ultimate arch-nemeses.** If you live with chronic illness long enough, "triggers" will become part of your regular vocabulary. There's the *inciting* trigger that typically coincides with your initial symptoms, and then there are the post-diagnosis party crashing triggers that can send your body into a full rebellion at random moments. For lupus patients and even some patients with psoriasis and eczema, sun and heat are two of the most common offenders— according to research published in *The Journal of Autoimmunity*,[2] about 70 to 80 percent of us deal with photosensitivity or heat-triggered symptoms.

With journaling, the pattern was undeniable. Five minutes in the Florida sun and, boom: fever, rash, sores, and a one-way ticket to Misery Island within hours. If I stayed out longer, that's when things got even more spicy: irregular heart rhythms, occasional hospital visits, and the beginning of a flare-up. My body basically screamed "We hate it here, Marisa!" every time I walked outside. So, after years of living like a vampire, I packed up my life and moved from Fort Lauderdale to the Canadian border in Upstate New York.

That drastic move was one of the best decisions I've ever made for my health. My body thrives in cold weather. I have the data, the journals, and the receipts to prove it. My flares were cut by more than half simply because the sun and heat weren't overwhelming me every day. I fully realize that not everyone wants to live in the arctic tundra alongside me, the snowplows, and an average of over 100 inches of snow per year—but that's the point. Some people feel *way* better in dry desert climates. Others love humidity or snow. It's divisive—Team Hot vs. Team Cold—but your body usually knows which team it plays for. So, listen to it, and pay attention to how your symptoms change during each calendar season. You might be surprised by improvements in symptoms when you let your body lead instead of forcing it to follow.

**Side note, my sun-sensitive friends:** Numerous autoimmune and chronic skin conditions—like rosacea, psoriasis, solar urticaria, atopic dermatitis, and xeroderma pigmentosum—can also come with a lovely bonus gift called *photosensitivity*. A real BOGO, if you will. And here's the kicker: it's not just the sun we have to worry about. UV light from indoor sources (looking at you, fluorescent office bulbs, tanning beds, and halogens) can trigger reactions as well.

If you're suddenly feeling feverish, rashy, or flare-y after sitting under bright lights at work all day, write it down in your journal and look for patterns. And don't worry—we're going to talk about workplace accommodations later, because no one should have to choose between a paycheck and their skin trying to spontaneously combust.

**Emotions played an intimate role in my physical symptoms.** Every major emotional surge I endured (sadness, stress, anger, anxiety—pick a flavor) came with a physical fallout within twenty-four hours. Once my nervous system flipped into high alert, it was like a full-body revolt: fevers, rashes, mouth sores, exhaustion, inflammation—an unwanted symphony conducted by cortisol and chaos.

When my grandmother—the woman who raised me—passed away, it completely shattered me. Within twenty-four hours, I spiraled into one of the worst flares of my life, one that put me in the hospital and lasted many months. Years later, when my father died, the same thing happened again. Same pattern, different flare, new tacky hospital bracelet. Guess what? It wasn't just the "big" losses—sometimes even lesser emotional shake-ups triggered a reaction. My journal was basically screaming the truth: Marisa, grief and stress physically affect your already exhausted immune system!

You might be curious about the science behind all of this: Basically, emotional stress activates the nervous system and floods the body with inflammatory chemicals. In a typical body, it's a nuisance. But "healthies" can combat the inflammation and come back to homeostasis. In a chronically ill body, it's gasoline on a brushfire. This realization from my journal pages changed everything for me. I started guarding myself differently on emotionally heavy days—doubling down on rest, staying consistent with or sometimes ramping up meds and supplements, and proactively using tools I was learning in therapy. I had to find ways to move emotions through my body, not store them like I had been doing for most of my life.

So, as a reminder when you're journaling, don't just track food, symptoms, activities or weather.

Track your heart.

Track the meltdowns, the breakthroughs, the bursts of grief, the spirals—and even your happy-cry moments, like weddings or babies or sappy commercials that catch you off guard. You may start to see exactly what I did: Your emotional world and your physical world are dance partners—and sometimes, your body is following the emotional lead.

**The foods I was choosing had quite an impact.** I always considered myself a healthy eater—and even more so after my diagnosis—devouring fruits and vegetables and making almost every meal from scratch with fresh ingredients. So, why did I feel terrible after so many meals? Turns out, I was unknowingly eating foods my body absolutely despised. Who knew? (Apparently, my allergist did.)

After a battery of blood and skin tests, she spilled the beans: Several of my "healthy staples" were wreaking havoc on my digestive system. I had food sensitivities to some and straight up food allergies to others. Apparently, having a higher incidence of allergies once you are diagnosed with certain chronic illnesses isn't uncommon, and vice versa. In fact, research shows that people with autoimmune disease have higher rates of allergic reactions.[3] In a study by The University of Birmingham, researchers discovered that people with allergies have elevated long-term risk of developing autoimmune diseases.[4] Additionally, a pediatric review highlighted that allergic diseases frequently co-occur with some chronic conditions, for example, asthma, atopic dermatitis, celiac disease, type 1 diabetes, and juvenile idiopathic arthritis often appear together, with these patterns suggesting lifelong immune dysregulation.[5]

For me, the biggest culinary betrayal? Avocados. My beloved, daily avocados. I ate them raw, baked them with eggs, used them in place of mayo and even made chocolate pudding out of them. Turns out several fruits and vegetables I ate often also came up high on sensitivity tests. Once I knew my trigger foods, I worked with a nutritionist to build a customized meal plan full of "safe foods," and—thanks to my allergist—slowly reintroduced some of the borderline ones. I'm still salty about avocados, though.

In today's world, you can't get through a quick social media scroll without seeing posts about another "miracle diet" or recipe guaranteed to fix everything from fatigue to frizz. And while some of these recipes and meal plans might be the epitome of "healthy" and may help with certain ailments or symptoms, if you have a food sensitivity or allergy to anything used in the recipe, you could be setting yourself up for additional issues and could be moving in the direction opposite to healing. I urge anyone living with a chronic illness to get proper allergy testing and, if possible, see a nutritionist afterward. These are essential tools needed to build your personal food blueprint—your own custom grocery list, meal plan, and recipe lineup that supports your body, sensitivities, and health conditions, not someone else's algorithm.

## Your 15–18 Minutes Starts Now

Let's pretend the day you've been waiting for is finally here. *The* appointment, folks. And in many instances, with the current state of our health-care system, you've likely waited weeks or even months for this appointment. On these days, I want you to think of your doctor's appointment as a high-stakes business meeting. You wouldn't walk into a job interview without intimately knowing your resume and experience from top to bottom, right? And you wouldn't walk into a business consultation or negotiation without arming yourself with research, would you? Well, similarly, don't stroll into the doctor's office like you're meeting a friend for brunch.

This is game time.

We want to make sure we have done our homework beforehand and have brought the necessary information with us. Be concise, but thorough—this isn't the place for a Netflix-style ten-episode recap of your entire health history as we only have a short amount of time. But remember, you're not just a patient; you're the CEO of your own health empire.

All that said, here's what I really want you to take away from this conversation: Journaling and tracking aren't just tools for your medical team—they're powerful tools for *you*. Through this practice, you'll get to know your body on an intimate level and bring doctors a clearer picture of what's actually happening. But there is also this truth: Even with all that data, it doesn't guarantee the doctor will "get it," take it seriously, or land on a diagnosis right then and there (wouldn't that be nice?). Think of your journal as a bridge—one that brings you a step closer to answers and a deeper understanding of your own patterns.

Even now, many years after my lupus diagnosis, I still journal on a regular basis. It helps me empty all the noise swirling in my head and notice when something new might be creeping in. It's become such a grounding and calming part of my life, I honestly can't imagine going a day without it.

## Getting the Right Tests and Referrals

Before we wrap up this chapter, there is one more topic I think is worthy of discussion. Time and time again, I hear from my fellow chronic illness warriors that even with data in hand, rehearsed conversations, and detailed questions, they feel they are not being heard when it comes to having the necessary tests conducted or referrals made. This is an issue dear to my heart because if any doctor I saw in those fifteen years of suffering had recognized something wasn't adding up and further tests should be done, my life may have taken a different path that didn't involve over a decade of anguish. I also remember what it feels like, especially just after my diagnosis, to leave a doctor's appointment and wish later on that day you had pushed for a certain test or referral to a specialist.

How many of us have heard the dreaded line: "Let's follow up in three to six months and see if things have gotten better."

Um . . . actually, *let's not.*

By the time we've dragged ourselves into that appointment, we're already running on fumes. The idea of waiting months while our bodies continue waving red flags is not just frustrating, it's unfair. The truth is, some tests can be ordered *today.* Some answers can start *now.*

Now, here's the thing: Doctors are human. They have blind spots, biases, and packed schedules. Maybe they just left an emotionally draining appointment and need a moment to focus. I get it. We all have off days. But here's what I also get—patients shouldn't have to keep showing up, repeating the same ol' story, only to leave with the same uncertainty, turn around months later, and repeat the cycle.

That's where your inner squeaky wheel comes in. And no, I don't mean going full "health-care Karen." This is about being firm but kind about what you need. You really do catch more bees with honey.

So, if through your research or say, speaking with a chronic illness advocate, you learn about a certain blood test or specialist that makes sense for what you're experiencing, speak up.

What if your doctor brushes you off? Honey, remember this: If your hairdresser hacked your bangs into oblivion, you wouldn't just smile and say, "Oh well, guess I'll live with this lopsided disaster for half a year. See you later!" You'd either ask them to fix it or find someone who could.

Your health deserves that same energy.

When you feel dismissed, you can try something along the lines of:

"I know you are extremely busy, but my symptoms are really affecting my daily life. Is there any reason we can't explore this further today?"

"I've been dealing with these symptoms for X (weeks, months, etc.) and I don't feel comfortable leaving here without some tests ordered so we can start finding answers."

And if you are feeling really bold and want to personalize your ask a bit more, you can state: "If it were your family member in this situation, would you recommend they wait, too?"

If you feel super uncomfortable even reading this, let alone saying it to a doctor, you're not the only one. But this can become less anxiety-producing in time; practice potential responses before your appointment using your own words so on game day, it will roll right off your tongue. Yes, this exercise might feel awkward but get in front of a mirror and repeat it until it feels natural and doesn't make you cringe.

Look, I get it. Speaking up to the White Coats can feel like trying to challenge your professor during class. We've been raised to believe that doctors sit at the top of the authority pyramid and questioning them is somehow disrespectful—or worse, dangerous. But here's the thing: Once your appointment is over, they go on to the next patient . . . and *you* are the one left living with every single minute of what was (or wasn't) decided in that room.

Yes, doctors undoubtedly deserve our kindness and respect—but so do *we*. Your health is not a one-way street. It deserves a two-way conversation. You are the CEO of your body and your voice belongs at the decision-making table.

Period.

I've noticed something else over the years: When I walk into an appointment prepared, with notes, questions, and a little "I'm-sweet-but-don't-you-dare-gaslight-me" energy, the tone shifts. Medical professionals seem to take me more seriously, dismiss me less, and, what do you know, the ball actually starts rolling a lot faster.

So, here's my best advice: Educate yourself like your life depends on it because, honestly, it does. Jump into different online communities like Instagram, TikTok, Reddit, or patient groups on Facebook and start connecting with people who get it. I have found this to be true: The chronic illness community is one of the most generous corners of the internet. People in these communities are thrilled to share what tests helped them, which doctors finally listened, or how they pieced their diagnosis together.

So, get in there and start asking questions. Gather stories. Compare notes. Then take what resonates into your next doctor's appointment.

Here's my final pro-tip for this chapter: If you do not have a primary doctor or family doctor, if you live in a rural community with limited medical professionals, or if you feel you are getting nowhere with your current medical team, there are numerous websites and companies today that let you order lab tests without a formal/

in-person doctor's appointment. I am not affiliated with these sites in any way but here are a few to consider:

- Walkinlab.com,
- PrivateMDLabs.com,
- LabCorp on Demand,
- Healthlabs.com
- Quest Diagnostics

That's right—DIY diagnostics are a thing now. It's like Instacart but for your blood. You can also search "websites that let you order blood tests without a doctor" on your internet browser and you'll find a plethora of other options. These services can become your new bestie if you are having trouble finding a primary doctor, are being dismissed, your doctor won't do further testing, or if you want to be proactive and have some testing done in advance of an initial appointment. To be clear, on-demand blood lab tests are generally not covered by insurance, as they are considered "self-initiated" wellness checks; you may have to take it slow with testing depending on your budget. Also, it's helpful to know that some of these online lab request companies allow you to pay via your HAS/FSA dollars.

At the end of the day, this chapter isn't just about data, journaling, or speaking up, it's about reclaiming our power in a medical system that can sometimes let us down. Remember: You are your body's best narrator. Every note you take, every symptom you track, every brave question you ask in a medical setting, trust me, it is all building upon one another. These aren't just tools; they're acts of love for a body that is trying so hard to fight for you.

## CHAPTER 5

# THE CHRONIC ILLNESS RELATIONSHIP AUDIT

Relationships change after a diagnosis and there's no cute card from Hallmark to ease the sting. I wish this truth didn't exist but here we are. Chronic illness has a knack for infiltrating every relationship we hold dear: family, friends, even that bestie who once swore she'd Thelma and Louise it with you (minus the cliff part, obviously). It tugs at the seams of the relational cloth, testing the stitching. Some seams rip and the fabric never quite lines up again, while others pull tighter, strengthened by the very strain meant to break them.

This chapter might feel a little messy and emotional—you'll likely have an "ouch" moment or two, maybe even a "Marisa, are you spying on my life?" sigh. But before you grab your tissues or Google "How to become a hermit in a tiny house on the Oregon coast," take a deep breath. There's still so much good here, even in the hard relational stuff.

Truth moment: Illness tilts a family's axis. Roles shift with zero to little warning. Children grow up faster than they should, and partners walk that weird line between lover and caregiver. But beneath the role reversals and shifts is something tender: love in motion, real and unvarnished, showing up even when no one knows quite what to do.

After more than twenty years since my diagnosis, I've learned this: Illness is a Renaissance-level master sculptor. It will carve out and reveal who can stand in the storm and who only wanted to be present on the sunny, picture-perfect Instagrammable days. Some relationships will crumble and yes, it will hurt your heart, but others will root deeper, becoming unshakeable in ways only hardship can forge.

Chronic illness doesn't just rattle the body: It exposes the heart. Sometimes you'll look at a loved one, thinking, *Who are you?* Other times, you'll watch people quietly drift away while you're left with memories and so many questions. Been there. Ugly-cried there. But this chapter on relationships isn't about blame or shutting out the entire world because of a diagnosis. It's about understanding how illness reshapes connection, what we can give, what we need, how people show up for us, and what we should no longer tolerate.

And here's the hopeful part of this conversation: Even if a diagnosis has impacted your relationships in a difficult way, you *will* laugh again. Joy will find you in the weirdest, most unexpected places. Peace will eventually inch its way back into your atmosphere. Because chronic illness is one of life's greatest juxtapositions: shrinking your world while expanding the depth of it at the same time. It unravels you just enough to help you rebuild with stronger boundaries, a softer heart, greater self-awareness and self-love, and a clearer understanding of who truly belongs in your life.

And, contrary to what we may think when we are in the thick of it, some people *will* stay—unyielding, loyal, and so beautifully human. And those who drift away? Well, maybe life is clearing space for the ones who are truly meant to walk beside you through the flares, the laughter, the late-night ER visits, the "can you help me wash my hair?" days, and everything in between.

## Family Ties

Some of chronic illnesses' most powerful shifts happen in the family dynamic, so let's start here. Because when chronic illness walks through the front door, it doesn't tip-toe in and hide in the corner—it shakes the very walls of family life. The person who was "fine" has to learn a new version of themselves and everyone else is often just as bewildered. Some family members rally like superheroes, armed with ice packs, CBD cream, and meal trains; others retreat in anger, confusion, or complete denial. It's messy, puzzling, and at times downright lonely.

And perhaps one of the most challenging plot twists in family life after a diagnosis is what I lovingly (and not-so-lovingly) call *the Ghost of the Old You.* It's that version of yourself who could do *All. The. Things*, effortlessly, energetically, and without ever needing a nap. If you're early in your chronic illness journey, you might not have a solid handle on any of this yet. You may very well be trying to prove to everyone and yourself that you can still do it all while also trying to figure out triggers, medications, side effects, and why your body suddenly behaves like the mean girl from your high school. But I promise—in time you will discover your new normal.

Where the Ghost of the Old You *really* likes to cause chaos is in family roles. Suddenly, your energy levels aren't just "different"—they are literally nonexistent. Symptoms hijack your plans. Tasks you knocked out in minutes before breakfast now feel like Olympic-level events. Cleaning, cooking, working, homeschooling, simply *existing* without needing a nap, even taking a shower suddenly takes enormous effort. And yes . . . this is where grief about how illness is affecting your family life enters the chat.

I know the word *grief* can feel heavy, but hear me out. Personally, I don't associate grief strictly with tragedy the way society can sometimes frame it. Grief is layered, complex, and, dare I say, transformational. It's a mix of heartbreaking and strangely beautiful because it reshapes you in ways you never intended but sometimes desperately needed.

When it comes to chronic illness, mourning certain family dynamics can show up in so many layers. One of the big layers of the grief onion is not operating the way you once did. Your partner may or may not understand that your daily checklist now has to be shorter or perhaps operate at a slower pace. What you used to get done in a day may take a week. Your partner may have to take on more responsibilities or a second job, as financial strain enters the picture if you're unable to work. Then there is the layer of how illness changes the lives of our children—and man, are children observant—wondering why you tire more easily, why sunshine suddenly means "danger" to mom or dad, or why every family outing now seems to involve a doctor's office.

And let's not forget the cultural and generational curveballs that get thrown our way. Phew, talk about some landmines! This is where guilt, tension, and unsolicited commentary from parents or in-laws often come marching in. Depending on your background, there may be deeply rooted expectations—expectations so rigid they leave absolutely no space for chronic illness to exist, let alone be accommodated or discussed in any way.

So, what do you do when it feels like sandbag after sandbag of guilt, worry, and grief is being stacked on your shoulders? The truth is, there's no one-size-fits-all answer here. Each of you reading this is navigating a different "new normal" and walking a path that is unique. But I *do* have a framework that can help you carve that path of grief and evolving family dynamics with a little more clarity and a lot more self-compassion.

Here's what I have discovered: Naming the grief as it pertains to changes in the family unit is one of the most powerful things you can do.

After naming what I am grieving, I then pair it with a strategy. Start by taking a few minutes to reflect and identify exactly what you're mourning in this moment and give it a name, whether that is out loud, on paper, screaming it into your pillow—you do you, babe. Maybe it's the health you once had, the loss of stamina, missing weekend funfests with your kids. Maybe you are grieving the unplanned rerouting of your life. Or stepping away from a career you loved.

Once I name my grief, its heaviness over me lessens a bit. It stops feeling like a dark shadow lurking in my peripheral vision and it becomes something tangible, something I can actually work through. And after you've named yours using the exercise I mentioned above, it's time to apply a strategy to it. What do I mean? Let's say you're grieving lost energy and drowning in anxiety because your house is literally one pile of crap away from appearing in an episode of *Hoarders.* Call a short family meeting. Say something like, "I'm in a new season with limited energy and learning how to navigate all of the recent changes. I need help with dinner, school pickup, and laundry." Use your own words, your own tone, but let the message stand. Delegate and come up with a plan. And trust me, this is going to feel awkward as heck at first. Growth and change often do. But pairing emotional recognition with practical support is key to surviving evolving family dynamics after a diagnosis.

And here's a reminder: If naming what is breaking your heart and creating a strategy feels completely overwhelming, you don't have to do it alone.

Therapy, coaching, or a trusted faith leader can be lifelines. I've leaned on professionals during the hardest storms (career loss, chemo, body changes), and the tools they gave me were game changers. Pride and ego have no place here—let support be your soft, safe place to land.

## Generational and Culture/Custom Clashes

Grief about family dynamics is just one fun piece (sarcasm, clearly) of the chronic illness puzzle. There are also those awkward-but-crucial talks with family members who believe "pull yourself together" is legitimate medical advice. And these situations can be even more complex when generational and cultural beliefs on what chronic illness is or isn't enter the conversation.

Have your parents, in-laws, or extended family members ever had a puzzled look on their faces—the one that silently asks "Can't you just do things like you used to?" If so, please know this: I see you. You're not alone in experiencing that heartache. In listening to thousands of patients over the years, I honestly can't think of one who hasn't wrestled with a similar family-related disconnect at some point.

Part of the struggle in understanding sits in the generational divide itself. Our parents and grandparents came from an era where illness was something you pushed through, not something you talked about. You absolutely did *not* do that! Also, chronic illness, especially autoimmune disease, wasn't as prevalent or recognized then. And it certainly wasn't tested for or discussed even a fraction of what it is today. Pain was often met with stoicism, silence, or shame. The world they grew up in rewarded endurance, not vulnerability. So, when they see us needing to rest, saying no, or choosing self-preservation over performance, it challenges the framework they've always known.

But here's the reality: Reworking your life to your body's current challenges, wanting to talk openly about what is happening, or seeking help through a counselor or faith counsel, is not a failure or weakness in any way. You are simply living by a new set of rules—ones that honor what your body requires to survive and even thrive within the limits your body has now set. And let me stress this, my friend, you are in no way weak for doing less or putting some things down during this season of your life. In fact, you are wise for doing what's necessary.

This is how you survive and ultimately thrive.

It helps to remember that family-members' reactions are often based in fear—fear of losing the version of you they once knew, fear of what they don't understand, fear of your mortality, or even fear that illness could touch them too. Sometimes, certain statements or questions may come wrapped in good intentions, but can land with a judgmental tone or air of disbelief. Which is why learning how to respond—with grace when possible and firm boundaries when needed—is essential to protecting your peace and your nervous system, which has a direct effect on your symptoms and overall health.

So, whether a loved one can't understand why you aren't hosting the holiday this year, why you can't eat a once beloved cultural delicacy, why you have cut down office hours or how many college credits you are juggling, or hell, even why you are taking your second nap by the afternoon and haven't washed your hair in six days, here are some ways to navigate those difficult moments.

These examples can help kick off a conversation and bridge the gap between generations and expectations, without losing yourself in the process. They range from gentle to firm and can be stated in verbiage you're comfortable with:

### *Gentle*

"I really appreciate your concern. I'm learning how to balance things so I can still be present, just in different ways."

"I love how much you want to help or include me. I'm learning how to find ways that work for my body and do not cost me days of recovery."

"I know I look healthy on the outside, but my energy comes in very limited amounts. I promise I'm not being lazy—I'm managing carefully."

"I understand this must feel strange for you to see me slowing down and navigating life differently. But I'm learning to live in a body that has new limits now."

"I still want to be part of things—it just might look a little different than before. I'm in a season where I have to limit what I say 'yes' to in order to care for myself."

"I know you're used to me showing up in a certain way in the past, but I'm doing my best to find a new rhythm that works for my health and energy levels."

### *Firm*

"I can't do everything I used to, and this is not up for debate or questioning. I'm learning to respect my body post-diagnosis, and need others to do the same."

"I understand that resting or napping might look like weakness to you, but it's actually what keeps me functioning."

"I know you mean well, but comparing me to who I 'used to be' isn't helpful. I'm doing my best with the challenges I am currently facing today."

"I will not continue defending my limitations. Believe me when I say 'no' or 'I am trying my best.'"

"I'm no longer available for conversations that question whether I'm trying hard enough. I'm always trying."

"When you dismiss my symptoms or expect me to 'get over it,' it makes me feel unseen. I need compassion, not condescension."

"If I decline an invitation or responsibility, it's not rejection—it's thoughtfully planning what my body can maintain for its survival."

"This is my new normal. I'd love your support as I navigate it, even if it looks different than what you expected."

Perhaps some resonated with you. Perhaps some made you feel downright uneasy as you read them. That's perfectly okay; we were never taught how to have these conversations, and we surely never thought we'd be in a position where we needed to have them! What matters is finding language that feels true to *you.* Whether you approach the situation with the gentleness of a cloud or the firmness of a brick wall, you are laying the groundwork of teaching the people around you how to treat, love, support, and show up for the new version of you that is here, trying every single day, and who is still worthy of love and grace.

## Navigating When Children Are Involved

Now, if parenting were a sport, chronic illness is most definitely the curveball that unexpectedly hits you smack in the face. If adult relationships aren't tricky enough when commingled with a chronic illness, we also have to figure out how to help our children understand. Yeehaw! Many parents I've spoken to over the years have said their children have taken these life changes in stride compared to other family members. Now, that's not to say that challenges don't exist, but they usually differ depending on the age group. And while raising children while also walking the chronic illness journey is not for the faint of heart, there is a beautiful element to the experience: You have a unique opportunity to teach your children about empathy, patience, and resilience, while modeling what it looks like to ask for help, receive help, and stick it out even when life gets messy.

### *Babies*

If your diagnosis arrived after childbirth, which is sadly, a common trigger for autoimmune and other chronic conditions, you're juggling grief and newborn wonder at the same time—which is unfair and brutal. My heart goes out to you. All you want to do is soak in those snuggles, but you may instead find yourself wondering: *Do I even have enough energy to lift this tiny human?* The exhaustion is real. And the guilt? Even worse. But I want you to know, while it won't be easy, you can still build a beautiful bond with your baby, even in this season of chaos. It will probably look a wee bit different than you imagined, but it can be just as rich.

In this season, small daily shifts can be the difference between overwhelm and stability. Tag-team with your partner, parents, or friends so you're not trying to be Superwoman on fumes. There is a reason they say to put the oxygen mask on yourself first. If energy or muscle fatigue is present, get creative; set up "command centers" around the house (think diapers, snacks, onesies, and wipes) to save needless trips and consolidate energy. This is especially helpful if you live in a multi-story dwelling. Communicate openly regarding your limitations and create a plan with your partner or family that allows you to take on more of the emotional connection tasks—like voice soothing, reading, or skin-on-skin snuggles—while they handle the more physical tasks.

Your situation will inform the solutions, but here are practical ideas to try as you find your groove:

1. **Supportive Gear is Your Friend:** Illness drains energy and often brings body pain and/or muscle fatigue, so lean into tools that make life easier. Swaddles, slings, adjustable bassinets, and front-opening tops or jumpsuits can relieve strain on your back and joints. Think of them not as "extras," but as essential survival tools in your thriving-with-chronic-illness toolbox.
2. **Make the Most of Floor Time:** Maybe a stroll around the neighborhood isn't in the cards today, but the floor can be just as magical. Spread out a blanket and sing, make silly faces, offer a gentle baby massage, or just breathe together. Capture these tiny moments in photos or short videos—they become powerful reminders on hard days when it feels like life is moving without you.
3. **Redefine What "Being There" Means:** Babies don't care if your home looks Pinterest-perfect or if you did your makeup. What matters is the connection. Sitting with them on your lap while someone else feeds them is still bonding. These quiet, simple moments are where the real memories live.
4. **Implement Routine Emotional Check-Ins:** Whether it's with your partner, trusted family member, or your therapist, regularly discuss what you are feeling, whether it's fear, anxiety or pressure. Saying it out loud keeps it from

consuming you and opens up clearer conversations about how you can be supported. If you're single-parenting, these check-ins help you see where boundaries and support systems are needed.

Even if your energy meter isn't what it was pre-pregnancy, there are still ways to stay deeply connected to your baby. Remind yourself often: Your child isn't measuring your love by how many times you pick them up or how clean the house is. Love grows through your presence, the beating of your heartbeat against their body, your smell, your gentle touch, and those small, special moments that just involve being, not doing.

### *Young Children/Pre-Teens*

Parenting young children and pre-teens while living with a chronic illness is deserving of its own medal ceremony. Seriously. This age group is all boundless energy, endless questions, and eagle-eye observation skills. They may not say it out loud, but they notice every shift. They can tell when dad or mom doesn't have the energy they used to or when playtime seems to get shorter and shorter. And because this is the age when curiosity skyrockets, gentle, age-appropriate honesty becomes essential. You don't need to deliver a TED Talk on your diagnosis, but a simple, truthful conversation can ease fears and help them understand what's going on. Look for children's books or movies you can read or watch together where chronic illness is part of the plotline, and give them an opportunity to ask questions.

Here are a few potential conversation starters when the time comes to have "the conversation:"

1. Mom/Dad's body has a limited energy level. Like your tablet, my 'battery' runs low and naps are my 'charging time.'
2. My illness is kind of like the weather—some days are stormy and I have to stay inside and rest more, and some days are sunny and I can do more with you.
3. My medicine is like tiny superheroes working hard inside me. Sometimes their big job makes me extra tired.
4. Think of my illness as a puzzle my doctors and I are trying to solve together.
5. Sometimes my body feels strong and other times it is tired and achy. You cannot catch this, and it isn't because of anything you did. Resting helps me maintain balance so I can hopefully have more "good" days.

Talking to your child about your illness is important—but conversation is only one part. Connecting, bonding, and curating joy together matters just as much. Here are a few ideas to make that happen:

**Create cozy, low-energy playtime:** Skip beach day and make the most of your living room. Let creativity lead and do art at the table, couch coloring sessions, puzzles or LEGO, and storytime picnics on the floor.

1. **Empowering tasks:** Kids feel safer when they feel useful. Let them choose the movie, be your snack chef, bring your water, or fluff your pillow—each a small helpful task framed as *trust*, not burden. Kids *love* purposeful responsibility.
2. **Create a "flare day" plan:** Prep ultra-low-energy activities for really tough days that include a special movie list perhaps played for your child on a tablet through headphones,

allowing you quiet time, special occasion snacks, and "quiet-time challenges" that work for your family.

3. **Bond through rituals:** Morning time not your easiest time of day? Same. Maybe these become the Saturday or Sunday morning-story time snuggle moments. A good friend of mine who is chronically ill, uses these snuggle-in-bed mornings for her kids to share three things: a happy moment of the week, a hard moment of the week, and who was their hero that week. If you need a nighttime idea, grab a blanket and stargaze together. Download a constellation app and explore the sky as a team.
4. **Start a weekly show-and-tell:** If you're couch-bound by evening, have your kids pick something new they learned each week and share it with you—a video, a fact, a cool story—while you rest beside them.

Simply put, young kids don't need endless energy from you. They need gentle explanations that make them feel safe, and they need presence far more than performance. Sacred moments, unhurried activities, snuggles and honest conversations are where the best memories can be made.

### *Teenagers+*

Anyone raising a teen—chronic illness or not—deserves a standing ovation. Teens come with big opinions, bigger hormones, and a world-class ability to slam every door they pass. Parenting through that *and* managing a chronic illness while watching your teen push for independence, privacy, and identity? Take a bow, you badass.

The good news: Teens are far more perceptive and empathetic than we often give them credit for. They notice even the most subtle shifts at home, even if they pretend not to. This is a season when open, honest dialogue matters, along with respecting their space and avoiding overwhelm or sugarcoating. There's still plenty of room for connection, communication, and genuine bonding, even if most of it happens between eyerolls and sighs. Here are some practical tips to make this stage survivable and meaningful:

1. **Let them be involved . . . on their own terms:** Most teens like responsibility when it feels like choice or teamwork, not obligation. If you need extra help during low-energy days, brainstorm together. Maybe they make dinner once a week, feed the dog, or take over loading the dishwasher.
2. **Make communication casual, not clinical:** Skip the anxiety-producing "let's sit at the table and talk" routine—it's basically teen-repellent at this point. Instead, try a late-night snack run, beach drive, or coffee/milkshake trip. Teens open up in neutral, low-pressure environments where the conversation unfolds naturally.
3. **Normalize their grief:** You aren't the only one grieving your health challenges. And your teen might feel angry, sad, frustrated and withdrawn, and not truly understand it is rooted in grief or anxiety about what may happen to mom or dad. It's important to help them understand it is okay to feel this way. To process the changes in family dynamics or witness a parent's health decline, a helpful option may be finding a neutral therapist, counselor, or faith-based leader who can help them process everything.

4. **Reimagine family traditions:** If Saturday night family dinners feel overwhelming, especially during a flare season, get creative: make it a "cereal and movie night" or "Uber eats, pajamas at 6 p.m. and puzzle night." In time, these can become your new normal. Consistency—no perfection—is what helps teens feel secure when life changes fast.

Conversation starters for talking about illness with your teen:

"I know things look different since I became ill. My symptoms might change our plans or responsibilities, and I know that can feel confusing or frustrating. It's okay to feel that way; I do too. I want you to know you didn't cause this and you don't have to fix it. Just tell me when it feels heavy so we can figure it out together."

"I want you to understand what's been happening with my body, not to scare you but to help things make sense. Some days will be easier for me; others may be tough. If it ever feels overwhelming, I'm here. You don't have to pretend you're fine; we have space for all of our feelings, and we'll adapt in time and get through this together."

Whether you are parenting a snuggly newborn, a never-tired grade-schooler, or a teen who only communicates via SnapChat messages and grunts, remind yourself that while chronic illness may reshape your family life, it won't steal the very heart of it. With creativity, love, and a lot of grace (for all involved), your family can feel stronger and more bonded than ever before, not in spite of your illness, but through it.

## Friendships

Friendships have been one of the most beautiful aspects of my chronic illness journey. On this road, I have found the people I never knew I needed—ones who don't flinch when I mention illness or a limitation that prevents me from taking part in something, and a family that accepts who I am today, sometimes in ways my own blood family cannot. I have found them to be the most generous, empathetic, fierce, and understanding people; some are also chronically ill, some are healthy, but they all understand my need to budget my energy and understand a "no" to an event isn't rejection but survival at times.

That's not to say I haven't had some friendships crumble under the weight of my diagnosis and how my lifestyle and schedule radically changed, especially when I was first diagnosed. These were people who knew my coffee order, my dark sense of humor, and how I'd spin a dozen plates without blinking. Those losses stung and required a grieving period.

If you notice a slow decline in communication, ongoing misunderstandings when you have to cancel plans, and eventually certain people detaching from your life after a diagnosis, I say this: Allow yourself to feel that ache. Just because you two are no longer traveling the same terrain on this journey of life, doesn't erase the love and bond you once shared. I'd also encourage you to not close yourself off to the possibility of meeting new ride-or-dies in the most unlikely of places in the future. Whether it is an online support group at three in the morning when the steroids are making sleep impossible, the person who sits in the chair beside you at the infusion center, or the neighbor who brings you groceries without being asked, life has a strange and miraculous way of bringing us the people we need.

In this new normal of life, you'll likely come to find your friendships will be filled with more honesty and intention. You'll desire quality over quantity, and gravitate toward people who are curious and empathetic, celebrate your small wins, and consider a fun Friday night watching a movie on the couch or playing a boardgame. There are good people out there, ones who will understand your boundaries, limitations, energy fluctuations, and everything else that comes with chronic illness.

And in the moments when life feels heavy, whether it's just post-diagnosis or during a major flare, and you can't piece together the right words but want to share what is happening with a friend, here are some examples to help your words take shape:

1. "Hey, I wanted you to hear this from me: I was diagnosed with (insert condition). It's been a lot to process. Some days are great and others are challenging. I adore our friendship and want you to understand sometimes it may be low-key, but your presence is so important to me."
2. "I wanted to keep you in the loop because you're important to me. I was diagnosed with (insert condition) and while I am learning to manage it, my energy and availability might look different than in the past. I appreciate patience while I am trying to figure this out."
3. "I'm sharing something personal with you—not for pity but to keep you in the loop. I was diagnosed with (chronic condition) and it is affecting my schedule and energy levels. Thanks for being someone I can share this with."

Now, I can't wrap up this section on friendship without some clap-backs for the people who just don't understand or don't want to even put in the effort to try (unfortunately, they exist). You might be dumbfounded or at a loss for words with how insensitive and hurtful humans can be at times. Hopefully these statements can be a springboard for ways to respond, though I am a strong believer in no response being a response:

1. "When you question my symptoms or how hard I am trying, it makes me feel unsupported. I need belief, not doubt in this season."
2. "This illness changed my life. I'm asking you to adjust with me instead of judging me for the limits I didn't choose."
3. "Trust me, if there were a 'try harder and be magically cured' button, I would've hit it approximately 500 times by now."
4. "Your comments are making an already hard situation harder. I need kindness from the people closest to me."

Whatever relationship we navigate after a diagnosis, we all learn the strange alchemy of illness in time. The one that burns away the performative and conditional ties and leaves us with those people in our lives who are saturated in empathy and understanding.

Relationships + chronic illness = different, not less. Show up for the ones that nourish you, set boundaries with the ones that don't, but never forget you are not walking this path alone. You have the opportunity right now to build the tribe that will carry you through this life. The question is, who will make the cut?

## CHAPTER 6

# LOVE (AND SEX) IN THE TIME OF ~~CHOLERA~~ CHRONIC ILLNESS

L.O.V.E. Ah, the four-letter word almost everyone is searching for. We are bombarded by it daily through songs, lovey-dovey social media posts, greeting cards, and couples who should *really get a room.* And because it is elusive, tricky, and already complicated enough to find, nurture, and sustain on its own, adding chronic illness to the equation makes for a plot twist even Colleen Hoover couldn't write (just kidding, I'm obsessed with her, btw!).

The reality is, love can get a little strange when your body is in full rebellion. But even in that messy and vulnerable space that is chronic illness, love can still show up. Whether you are dating after a diagnosis, adjusting to shifts in your existing relationship after your health did an unexpected backflip, grieving a love lost because a diagnosis came barreling through, or just want creative tips on keeping the spark and the communication alive when health challenges insist on third-wheeling it every night, you're in the right place.

Love looks different when your body and your health change. In its purest form, love will stretch, bend, pause, wait patiently, adapt, and carry you as you navigate what feels like a rollercoaster of chaos. Yet chronic illness has this cruel way of whispering the exact opposite into your ears (and heart), making you question if experiencing real love post-diagnosis is even truly possible.

Quickly, the doubts and questions can start pouring in:

> Can someone actually love me sick?
> Who will want me if my body has changed so much?
> What if I can't do what I did in the past—physically, sexually, and emotionally?
> What if someone has to take care of me for a season?
> Why choose me when "healthy" options exist?

And those are just the tip of the iceberg.

The questions we contemplate at times are heavy and heartbreaking. Chronic illness can trigger insecurities we never knew existed, warp our self-image and confidence, and perhaps in one of its worst effects on our emotional health, convince us that because we are ill, we are less deserving of receiving love, intimacy and connection (this of course is one thousand percent untrue and we are still unequivocally worthy). I experienced this firsthand over twenty years ago and thought for sure I was destined to live alone forever with my dog and my plants.

But here's the beautiful and hope-filled truth: A diagnosis doesn't disqualify you from falling in love and experiencing love from another person. It doesn't cancel out the possibility of finding a forever partner who is willing to walk this journey with you, and it also doesn't mean intimacy, sex, communication, and spontaneity are forever exiled—they just might require a different approach, some creativity and a bit of flexibility (literally and figuratively).

Regardless of where you are on your romantic timeline, know there can still be so much goodness up ahead when it comes to matters of the heart. And with that, let's start where so many of us find ourselves at one point or another: dating and loving while chronically ill.

## The Dating Season

For all of you currently in the dating pool, you hold a special place in my heart. Dating is tough—even when two physically healthy people get together! Add in a chronic illness diagnosis and let's just say, things get really interesting. And while dating culture has transformed wildly since I was last in the arena decades ago (like apps, emojis, unsolicited photos, and people who think "wyd?" is a full conversation + foreplay!), some aspects have not changed drastically, like when and how it is best to disclose a health challenge.

I've heard every approach under the sun on this topic from my single friends. And while, if you ask a dozen people with chronic illness about this aspect of dating, you'll typically get double that number in responses, some clear patterns emerge (and interestingly enough are often tied to certain personality types, including):

1. **The "Let me observe for a while" crowd**: These guys and gals typically prefer a few solid dates to determine if there is potential for a serious relationship before opening up about a diagnosis. The logic here? If there is no potential for long-term commitment, why share something so intimate? There is also a deeper privacy and protection element here, meaning there's no reason to hand over your health information to someone

who may not stick around and possibly repeat it to others in the future.

2. **The "Lay it all on the table immediately" squad**: Ah yes, my people: the straight shooters who like to lay their cards on the table. This camp usually feels that if someone reacts poorly to the "I have X condition" conversation, *wonderful,* because that saves weeks or months of wasted energy and dashed hopes. The belief? If this conversation scares someone or immediately brings out red flag energy, then they are most likely not your long-term, romantic ride-or-die. And that is absolutely okay because it frees one up quickly to find the person who extends a hand rather than recoils or questions you when the word "illness" comes up.
3. **The "It's obvious from go" crew**: I've been a part of this crew more times than I can count back when I was dating (you know, when dinosaurs still roamed the earth). There was no way to keep it under wraps when an uproar of rashes and sores on my skin broke out, and/or I was using a walker or wheelchair. I feel this group has the unspoken advantage of the visual cue—so the conversation tends to happen naturally. And honestly? That visibility often filters out many of the wrong people from "go." Notice I use the word advantage above; if you were just diagnosed and have outwardly visible symptoms and/or you're not totally comfortable using mobility devices out in public yet, this might feel like a disadvantage. But think of it this way: If someone is turned off or uncomfortable with your reality out of the gate, isn't it better to know that right away?

The truth is, the "when to disclose" question doesn't have a one-size-fits-all answer because there is no "right time." There's only the right-for-you-time that aligns best with your situation, specific diagnosis, and personality. But no matter when you choose to have that conversation, there are ways to disclose the information in a less anxiety-producing way without vomiting your medical chart to someone. Here are some examples that may prove helpful:

### *In-Person Prompts*

**Lighthearted yet practical:** I'm navigating a plot twist called _______. I am managing it daily but it sometimes requires conserving my energy and making adjustments in my schedule . Just wanted to give you the synopsis before we get too invested in the full storyline.

**When you are feeling a deep connection after a few dates:** I'm really enjoying where this is going and because of that, I'd like to share something personal. I live with _______. It doesn't define who I am but it is a piece of my daily reality. If you have any questions about it, I'd be happy to answer them.

**Casual, first-date drop (if you feel led):** Hey, I wanted to mention something quick that is a part of my world. I live with a chronic illness and I am managing it but it does shape my daily life. I'm not looking for pity or solutions, just wanted to be honest before this gets deeper.

**When disclosure is unavoidable because of symptoms/mobility devices:** So, you have probably noticed X. And I'm totally okay! This is just part of my life. If you are curious and want to learn more about _______, I am happy to talk about it.

### *Brief Online Quips for Dating Profiles*

**Short and Sweet:** "Living with a chronic illness/autoimmune disease. Yes, I am a lot of fun. No, it's not contagious."

**Creative yet Empowered:** "Chronic illness warrior. This storyline has made me stronger, softer, and more intentional. If you like depth, kindness, and a slower pace, we will get along marvelously."

**Bold and high-confidence:** "I navigate life beautifully with a chronic illness. If empathy, patience, and compassion aren't in your toolbox, please move along."

Whether you are dipping a toe or reverse-somersault diving into the dating pool, it's essential to reflect on *when and how* to disclose your health information in a way that honors your situation and comfort level. That being said, we also need to talk about what happens after the conversation . . . because reactions can run the gamut of the response spectrum. Some people will be authentic and unshaken, seeing your health condition as just one of the many threads in the fabric of who you are. Sadly though, others might respond well in the moment—and even say all the right things—only to ghost you days or weeks after the conversation when reality sets in. And while they may genuinely believe you are an amazing person, they might realize they are not equipped—or honestly, even willing—to navigate the unpredictability of what chronic illness looks like.

This realization, which can brutally sting, doesn't make that person a villain and it certainly doesn't make you unlovable; what it does is clear space for people who are ready to show up for your life (ups, downs, and all of it), while helping you decide what you will/won't tolerate after disclosing your health information.

So, what should you look for after "the talk"? Whether it's a green light or a long string of bold red flags waving in your face, all these signals are worth paying attention to:

### *The Green Lights*

- Respond with statements such as "Thanks for trusting me with this information," or "I'm happy you felt comfortable enough to share this with me."
- Ask curious and respectful questions about the condition; ask how they can support you; ask what tangible ways you accept help, etc.
- Respond to adjustments in plans or schedules with flexibility and compassion, rather than annoyance, guilt or manipulation.
- Don't default to fix-it mode and subsequently get frustrated when you don't comply.
- Consistently show up, even on the difficult days, rather than making excuses.
- Aren't pushy and allow you to disclose difficult and/or traumatic health experiences on your timeframe.
- Actively make space for your needs, including planning dates around energy levels, temperature, and/or seating preferences, food allergies, ability to travel, accommodation needs, etc.
- Appreciate your *entire* being and understand illness is just one part of your story, not your whole identity.
- Is willing to learn more about the condition and actually follows through by researching resources and educating themselves.

### *The Red Flags*

- You notice early on a rewriting of your health experience by minimizing symptoms or acting as though they know your body better than you do. This may be a seed of future gaslighting.
- They purposely test your limits and/or don't believe aspects of your health condition. Examples may be forcing you to try food you are allergic to, working out or engaging in a physically demanding activity that is beyond your body's ability, or forcing you to stay out longer when you are exhausted.
- They want to be overly involved immediately, attending every appointment, playing a role in your treatment decisions, etc. Side note: These are great aspects with a long-term partner and can relieve so much stress on someone who is chronically ill. But . . . and it's a big but, when it is done at the very beginning of the dating stage, it might be a lovebombing signal and point to a person's desire to make you dependent on them. This could also potentially be used later as a manipulation and guilt tactic under the guise of "look how much I did for you." Just no.
- They become angry or frustrated when an unexpected health challenge, flare day, or fatigue interrupts plans. If you notice these inconveniences trigger irritation, sarcasm, or responses like door slamming or ghosting for days after the change in plans, please save yourself now. Trust me when I tell you this is going to get worse in time.
- They try to control your narrative by diagnosing what you are experiencing. Examples include, "You're not having

trouble breathing, it's just anxiety," or "There's nothing wrong with you, you just need to drink more water," or "You don't need to call an ambulance, you are overreacting." This isn't compassion or loving behavior on any level.

Some of the reg flags I mentioned might've hit a nerve and believe me, I understand. Even writing that list stirred up memories of my younger self, making me wish I could time travel and give her a hug and a serious but loving pow-wow. But back then, I didn't have the confidence I do now. Unfortunately, I believed that being sick equaled me being less than and that I should have been grateful if anyone wanted to be with me *at all.* Because of these untruths, I tolerated behaviors I didn't deserve and never should have allowed. I've grown so much since those days thanks to therapy, a growing faith, maturity, and a whole lot of boundary-building. I swear, today I am basically a professional red-flag sniffer!

But here is the really difficult conversation about red flags that needs to be had: They don't only show up on first or second dates or even in friendships. Some of you might have recognized red flag behaviors on that list in someone you've been with for a long time. Perhaps you have a home or children together. The relationship dynamic can get even more complicated when the mistreatment starts after your diagnosis, when you've already built a life with that person. Suddenly your entire world is not only turned upside down, but the person you rely on and trust the most isn't responding compassionately.

If this is the situation you are in right now, I want to gently say: You aren't being dramatic and you are not to blame. Chronic illness can sometimes magnify and tilt the power imbalance in a relationship, especially if that illness causes you to become more dependent physically, emotionally, or financially on someone. We become more vulnerable when dealing with a debilitating illness, whether it's physical or emotional vulnerability, isolation, financial strain, identity loss, confusion in navigating the health-care system, etc. Psychology coins this as "vulnerability stacking" and unfortunately, people who tend to be controlling or who display narcissistic tendencies can exploit these vulnerabilities.

Whether you've been dating someone for a week or ten years, if you feel belittled, unsafe, dismissed, isolated, pressured, or controlled via finances, these are not little quirks that may get better in time. These are often toxic and/or abusive behaviors and being diagnosed with a health challenge isn't an excuse for someone to treat you this way.

Your safety is what matters most. If any of the above resonates with you, please consider reaching out to a counselor, coach, or even a domestic-violence advocate. Doing so doesn't mean you have failed in some way. Doing so gives you the clarity and support you deserve and the ability to create a plan that protects your physical and emotional well-being. Professionals in this area can help you create step-by-step exit strategies that take your health, finances, mobility, and other limitations into consideration.

Please remember that getting a diagnosis doesn't diminish your value. You are still worthy of love, respect, and dignity and deserve to be in a relationship that is safe and that honors who you are—diagnosis and all.

### *Navigating Challenges in Long-Term Partnerships*

For those of you reading who are in a long-term relationship or marriage that got sideswiped by an unexpected diagnosis, you face a unique set of challenges as both you and your partner are trying to adjust to a new normal. As I've mentioned before, there is always a grieving season, and it isn't just you navigating this process. Both members of the relationship feel this shift and need to grieve the plans and the future you thought you'd have together. But not all plans and dreams have to be exiled and forgotten about. Instead, with communication and creativity, and two people determined to walk this path together without throwing in the towel because things may get bumpy up ahead, a meaningful life is still possible.

There is no easy roadmap here, as every relationship is different, but I will stress this: Communication will be your lifeline and your best friend. I'm talking about raw, challenging conversations filled with emotions and possibly discomfort followed by moments of unexpected connection and joy. One of the most important things I've learned navigating these waters in particular is this: Relationships fare better when both partners face the diagnosis as a united front, not as opponents. The two of you vs. the illness, not you vs. each other. I'm not saying all days will be rainbows and unicorns but relationships can still thrive despite the challenges of an illness.

As you begin to navigate the path post-diagnosis, you may feel shock and denial. Fear, anxiety, and an onslaught of questions may keep you awake at 3 a.m.:

How did this happen out of nowhere?
What does the future hold for us?
What if treatment doesn't work?
What if we can't afford our home/groceries/medication?
What if my partner doesn't want to be with someone who is sick?

For the person diagnosed, there may also be questions tied to one's identity that involve how their body and health might change if they will lose their ability to be independent or if illness will prevent them from working or taking care of children. Partners may be wrestling with feelings about their own identity shifting from lover to caregiver. And, at times, feelings of resentment or sadness may bubble up as life dreams hit pause for a season.

And if all of this isn't hard enough, let's not forget: Society doesn't make space or help couples navigate life when a chronic illness butts into their storyline. There's no drug store aisle filled with cute animal cards that share "Congrats on figuring out your medical mystery" or "Sorry your life just blew up" one-liners. And most employers of spouses aren't exactly lining up to give the partner some extended time off or work-at-home options while the couple get a handle on their new normal.

Society, the workforce, etc. is set up for able-bodied, healthy people and the world we live in barely scratches the surface in recognizing how much a relationship withstands when a diagnosis is thrown into the mix. The day-to-day shifts, recalibrations, and flexibility needed are monumental and almost impossible to understand if you have never experienced it first-hand.

So how can love withstand these seismic shifts?

Bottom line: It will be a daily decision to work together, communicate, and create a plan that has the flexibility built into it to allow for the moments the rug gets pulled from under your feet. Again, naming the "hard thing" that is happening at the moment together—whether it's delegating who can pick up the kids on flare days or how you can still have date night if you are unable to leave the house, and subsequently creating a strategy—can make it feel much more bearable.

Navigating a relationship alongside a chronic illness isn't easy, but that doesn't mean throwing in the towel is the better option. Historically and statistically, relationships suffer when a diagnosis enters the picture. Studies show on average that a marriage is seven times more likely to end if the woman becomes seriously ill vs. if the man becomes ill.[1] This is especially hard to wrap my brain around considering, according to research from The National Institute of Health (NIH), women are diagnosed with chronic health conditions more than men.[2]

This reality hurts.

But statistics don't write your story—you do. With intention, patience, and fierce love, plus the implementation of intentional strategies, we can keep our relationships intact and emerge from the storm even stronger. Here are a few to consider:

1. **Name the Hard Stuff:** Regularly call out what is difficult: from finances and lack of sleep, to rescheduling routines because of medical appointments, or the sudden lack of spontaneity. When it is called out, it doesn't feel so overwhelming and can be tackled or at least understood. Then, brainstorm what some potential solutions could be, such as simplifying, delegating, or even just pausing what is top priority right now. Sometimes there won't be a specific solution right at that moment. Some solutions take time to create as you both learn how illness truly affects your relationship routine.
2. **Exhibit Transparency**: If you are the person with the diagnosis, speak up. Trust me when I say it is not easy at all for others, even our partner, to understand how we may feel

decent one day and be bedridden the next day. Your partner is not a mind reader. Be as transparent, explicit, and clear as possible, and state your needs. Are you experiencing pain or fatigue? Don't assume they know you are struggling just by looking at you.

3. A friend of mine bought me a two-sided octopus plushie to help me better communicate. On one side, the plushie is smiling and if you turn it inside out, the octopus looks disheveled and pissed off. Without even saying a word sometimes, I use this to just let others in the house know, *today isn't the best day*. This strategy actually works best when both partners put it into practice. If you are the health partner, it's crucial to share your emotions and thoughts too. Everyone deserves to have their voice heard and by speaking out, less resentments and misunderstandings build up.
4. **Express Appreciation, Often**: The daily add-ons when living with chronic illness, such as pharmacy runs, shifting plans to fit in doctor appointments, or a partner taking on extra responsibilities, can make life feel transactional. Gratitude and appreciation create a connection and it is a two-way street. If you are the person with the diagnosis, express appreciation for your partner folding the laundry or the quick back rub they provided.
5. **Acknowledge how your partner's life has also changed** in many ways and offer a sincere thank you for their patience. On the flip side, the healthy person can also express appreciation to their partner. Acknowledge how special he/she is to you and remind him/her that a diagnosis doesn't change your love.

6. **Illness-Free Conversation Zones:** One of the most important things I learned in my marriage while chronically ill was the following: We all need personal time to enjoy a hobby or relax where our illness isn't mentioned or the focus. For me, this was always painting, writing, or watching Netflix with my girlfriends. In addition to alone time that doesn't get overshadowed by illness, you and your partner also need time together to create connectedness and closeness that doesn't involve driving to a medical appointment or having a conversation that involves health issues. I realized over the years that illness infiltrated every area of our life, so we needed specifically curated moments where we could just be and enjoy one another where illness wasn't the highlight or interrupter of our time together.
7. **Increase Your Ability to Be Flexible**: Over the past twenty years I have learned that illness throws curveballs. Flares, exhaustion, doctor appointments: All of it requires a flexibility muscle that needs daily stretching. For the person with the diagnosis, you may get annoyed that you aren't able to fit as many tasks into a day as you used to. For the partner, you may feel frustrated that extra responsibilities are falling on your shoulders. So how can you increase your ability to be flexible and let go of the guilt and shame game? Ask yourself: "Will the world fall apart if this doesn't get done today?" (Spoiler: it won't.) And then sincerely let that s*&% go.
8. **Keep Courting One Another:** Dating your partner should never stop, chronic illness or not. Maybe a major road trip isn't in the cards physically or financially but you can recreate

your favorite movie date-night at home with blankets, popcorn, and other favorite snacks by your side. Maybe courting in your relationship is writing quick love letters to each other occasionally or a random text that shares how they made you feel loved that week. Micro-dates are fun too: a five-minute slow dance before bed at night, a game of cards on the living room floor, or a short drive along the beach listening to your favorite tunes. There are so many ways to keep pursuing one another amid illness.

### Intimacy 101: "Let's Talk About Sex, Baby"

Now, let's have some real talk about a topic you are probably not mentioning at your doctor appointments: how chronic illness is crashing your intimacy game. Keeping a relationship alive can be challenging enough, but when chronic illness rolls into the party, intimacy and sex can sometimes shift to the bottom of our priority list. But intimacy is crucial for our mental and physical health, and is what sets a romantic partnership apart from every other relationship in our lives. So how do we continue to nurture this sacred part of our relationship when we feel like we are already drowning?

For starters, we have to consider ways to intentionally infuse our relationships with moments of connection. Both partners have to also accept that at times, for numerous reasons, actual penetrative sex is off the table (or bed, literally). This isn't as uncommon as you might think; in fact, research shows less sexual activity taking place in relationships where one person is ill, versus the general population.[3] This can occur due to physical pain, fatigue, side effects from medication, the psychological aspect of one's body, and/or weight changing because of treatments, depression, and even the relational dynamic that has shifted from partner to caregiver. And yet, despite how often a couple's sex and intimacy life is impacted due to illness, studies also show most health-care providers don't bring this up during appointments, so couples are left to figure it out on their own—and in the process, their intimacy life takes a hit.[4]

I've heard different versions of the same dilemma brought up time and again in support groups and late-night DM conversations. Story after story, women (and men, on rare occasions) let down their guard and share how rashes, weight gain or loss, sores, scars, hair loss, and an unexpected need to use mobility devices have completely upended their body image and self-confidence. Others grieve the loss of how they once felt in their bodies. Some have shared that they feel "broken" because they aren't the same person as when their partner married them. In these conversations, I've noticed common threads: exhaustion and stress causing low sex drives, libido taking a hit from a variety of new medications, and physical pain because of surgeries, dryness, etc. If any of these resonate with you, please know you are not alone in navigating these harsh realities.

Sustaining intimacy in the face of chronic illness requires reimagination and redefinition that can only be done by the two people involved. Intimacy is so much broader than sex; it can begin gently and simply, like reaching for your lover's hand while in the grocery store, a soft cuddle, teasing one another in the kitchen, or a light scalp or foot massage while sitting on the couch. It can be playful and humorous: a silly private joke, funny nicknames, and laughing at the absurdity that chronic illness can infuse into life at times. It's flirting and teasing and letting the other person know they still have your heart and it is just as much emotional as it is physical.

When the time comes for the act of physical touch, sex may not always be the end game. In fact, depending on your condition and the severity in this season, it may not be the end game for a while. And that is okay. There are other creative ways to give and receive pleasure that don't involve actual intercourse.

One tip that I always encourage is to remove the expectation that every sexual encounter has to look like it *used to* with your partner. We evolve, our lives change, our sexual desires and ways we receive love changes. An unexpected hug in the kitchen as you prepare dinner together that turns into a passionate, lengthy kiss can be fulfilling. I've learned that bringing yesterday's expectations into today's reality is a fast track to feeling frustrated and let down. What works instead? Flexibility, curiosity, and no-filter conversations from each party involved about pleasure, desire, and what actually feels good *right now.*

Now let's talk actual practical ideas—from sweet to highly sensual—no penetrative sex required:

1. **Slow Dancing at Home:** Dim the lights, cue your go-to romance song, and let nostalgia lead the way. Melt into one another and let your bodies lead the way, not in a performative way but for presence and closeness. If standing isn't an option, snuggle in bed and sway to the rhythm right where you are.
2. **Bubble Bath or Shower Ritual:** Light some candles, cue a sensual playlist, and soak together. Warm water, and even Epsom salts, soothes sore joints, and gentle massages can bring both relief and connection while adding a level of sensuality. Enjoying an interruption-free, intimate

conversation while the rest of the world disappears is a beautiful way to connect in the midst of life's chaos.

3. **Snuggles and Storytelling:** If it's a flare day and staying in bed is a must, skin on skin snuggles can release oxytocin, the bonding hormone, which helps increase feelings of romantic attachment and trust. While snuggling, take turns telling one another an imagined romantic or sensual story, or share a favorite sensual memory between the two of you, recalling moment by moment. This is a sure-fire, low impact, and no-pressure way to bond with your beloved. Add feather-light fingertip tracing along arms or back for extra effect.
4. **Elevated Pillow Talk:** Phones off, lights low, all electronics on "do not disturb." Connect with one another through words; talk about fantasies, what you find sexy, and how you've felt loved lately. Laugh, cry, flirt, get vulnerable—whatever brings you closer. Sometimes talking can be just as sensual and intimate as the physical act itself.
5. **"My Guided Touch" Game**: One partner guides the other's hand across their body, giving clear feedback on what feels good in terms of pressure, pace, and location. It's deeply intimate and erotic, empowering, and requires zero pressure for sex.
6. **One-way Self Touching**: If mutual participation isn't possible because of body pain or fatigue, you'd be amazed how sensual it is for one partner to pleasure themselves while the other watches, affirms verbally, gently touches them during the act, and provides a lot of eye contact. This shared experience can prove to be as equally intimate and pleasing as penetrative intercourse. Don't believe me? Try it tonight!

7. **Fantasy, Role Play, and Toys:** If your body's up for it, try a low-effort role play or read an erotic story aloud to each other. And don't feel ashamed to let toys be your helpers on the painful days, especially ones that are hands-free or require minimal effort. Sensuality doesn't have to be strenuous.

All romantic relationships take ongoing work and commitment to one another, even when everyone's healthy. When a diagnosis decides to butt in, it just means you need to amp up the creativity, patience, and communication.

Yes, life may be different than planned, but you are doing it together. As you learn how to navigate this chapter, a deeper bond and even deeper connection can occur. Love isn't defined by perfect timing and flawless bodies. When two people are willing to continue trying, despite the obstacles, despite the doctor's "diagnosis," despite the fact that we live in a society where relationships seem so disposable, the truth is, love *can* adapt and it can absolutely endure and thrive even when your health feels uncertain. Together, you're choosing love. One step, one conversation, one loving gesture, and one day at a time.

# CHAPTER 7

# REIMAGINING THE DAILY GRIND

Most people think of employment when they hear the term "daily grind." And while that isn't wrong, chronic illness gifts a bonus daily grind. Aren't we lucky? Because the truth is, managing a chronic illness is actually a full-time job in and of itself, one most healthy people will never understand unless they get their very own backstage pass. Managing doctor appointments, bloodwork, treatments, procedures, scans, side effects, rest days, medications, diet, alternative protocols, triggers . . . and a side of "Why is my immune system doing that now?" requires Herculean mental and physical energy from a body and mind already running on low battery.

So, how do we pair all of that while trying to maintain our careers? How do we juggle passions, responsibilities, ambitions, and the basic need to feed, house, and insure ourselves and our families on days when taking a shower feels like climbing Mt. Kilimanjaro in flip-flops?

Every single person diagnosed with a chronic illness will eventually face the same gut-punching questions on this topic:

Is working full-time possible for me, right now?
Can my body keep up with my employer's expectations?
What will happen to me and my family if I cannot work?
How do I balance work and the physical, emotional, and logistical demands of this illness that clearly doesn't respect my to-do list?

I was diagnosed at the very beginning of my career as a nurse, something I'd fought hard for through years of schooling, clinical rotations, exams, and pushing through symptoms I didn't yet understand. And then, *poof*. A diagnosis hit, my health collapsed, and the career I'd worked so hard for evaporated before my eyes. My days consisted of bouncing between hospital beds to my bedroom at home for almost three years. There was no way I could survive a twelve-to-fourteen-hour hospital nursing rotation, when I in fact had a nurse coming to my home to help me bathe. If you find yourself in a situation like this, my heart goes out to you; the emotional fallout is real, and the anxiety and questions multiply fast.

The reality is, many chronic illnesses are episodic and experience seasons of non-flares and flares. The unpredictability of when these flares hit, well, they are about as fun as the third wheel no one invited on your hot date. We often don't know how we'll feel when we wake up, so attendance, deadlines, productivity, and consistency can feel like a roulette wheel. And while remote work has become increasingly common post-COVID (possibly one of the very few positives from that pandemic), much of society still functions in a traditional 9–5 structure designed around those I call "the healthies," who have stable energy output and lots of predictability when it comes to their health. Many newly diagnosed people don't yet understand how flares truly impact them. So they try to perform exactly as they did pre-illness—hustling, pushing, overcommitting, and telling themselves they can "bounce back later." They still try to reliably produce the same output as they did previously, typically leading to a constant cycle of overdoing it, never fully recharging during downtime, and ultimately burning out or landing themselves in the hospital.

No one can sustain their old pace when they are chronically ill.

Trust me—I tried. I lost my career and nearly lost my life. I'm not saying you can't get back to a strong healthy version of you, but there are a lot of steps on that journey; more on that in later chapters.

While you may know in your heart (and by your joints and bones screaming at you daily) that continuing your previous work output feels impossible, the world (and internet) is shouting a different message: "Push Through! Keep Going! It Could be So Much Worse!" As if your entire life hasn't just been bulldozed by a diagnosis. And whether it is shame, pride, embarrassment, ego, or some desperate final attempt to appear "normal," "healthy," and "unchanged" to those around us, many of us push ourselves to the brink.

Eventually, keeping up the facade takes up more energy than the actual job (and yes, for my fellow Spoon Theorists: Maintaining the facade alone burns through half the cutlery drawer).[1] What we actually need is a moment of truth with ourselves; a deep internal audit of where our health currently stands and whether full- or part-time work is actually *safe* and *sustainable* for the body. When I say sustainable, I mean a career choice that supports us financially without requiring us to spend every day off recovering, adding new medical interventions just to stay afloat, or ping-ponging from one flare to the next because we're living in permanent overdrive.

And here's the kicker: A sustainable career choice is not a one-size-fits-all answer.

For some, it means changing career fields entirely. For others, it means becoming an entrepreneur and/or working fully remote. For others still, it means applying for disability because their body has staged a full-blown coup against basically everything. In the pages that follow, we'll figure out what the right choice looks like for you if your current role is no longer compatible with your health.

## Workplace Rights and Workplace Culture: The "Must-Have" Conversations

If your current full- or part-time job is manageable or you're stable enough to apply for new roles, we need to have three big "pow-wows". These revolve around: your legal rights, disclosure, and navigating workplace culture without losing your mind or your spirit.

### *Disclosure: Before Interviewing and After Accepting a Position*

Let's start with a question many people ask me online: "Am I legally obligated to disclose my chronic illness or disability during a job interview?"

The short answer? No.

The longer answer? Still, absolutely not. And in most circumstances employers typically aren't allowed to ask but there are some exceptions.

It's a divided camp when it comes to disclosing early on; some argue early disclosure builds trust and can help you determine if a potential employer seems supportive, whereas others believe it opens you up to quiet rejection. Personally, I've been in interviews where I felt certain I was a top candidate until, I suspect, someone Googled my name and landed in the middle of my chronic illness advocacy universe. Surprise! Chronic illness is not always the crowd-pleaser. The truth is, rejection may very well happen if you disclose early on. And no, the employer will never use *that* as the reason you were passed over, because *it is illegal.* So, you will often receive a vague "We've moved in a different direction" email.

Because I have had this happen upon early disclosure, I flipped my own script. Instead of hiding my reality, I began sharing my limitations alongside my track record of what I've accomplished *despite* them. That transparency paints me as steady, accountable, dedicated, and adaptable and often opens the exact doors meant for me.

That being said, you must do what is right for you in the season you are in. Remember, during initial interviews, health and disability questions from employers are typically off-limits, though in most online job applications, an area asking applicants to "voluntarily" disclose disability status may appear. If you feel questions during your interview are leaning in the direction of personal health and disability status, redirect the employer to your abilities and experience.

Now, here is an important nugget: If you need a reasonable accommodation to perform the essential functions of your job, then you are required to disclose a disability or health condition. No, you don't have to dim the lights, put on a top hat and spill out an entire TED talk on your health journey. You simply name the limitation and the accommodation needed and explain how it supports your ability to perform the job. You can also shift the focus to how these accommodations have positively worked for you in the past, if applicable.

## *Accommodations, the ADA, and Your Legal Rights*

So, now that we have said the magic word—accommodations—let's break down what this actually means in real life. We'll begin with a quick refresher on the Americans with Disabilities Act (ADA). Simply put, the ADA is a federal law that prohibits discrimination against people with disabilities and chronic health conditions and requires employers to provide reasonable accommodations so employees can perform their job functions. If you've never learned about the "Capitol Crawl," go look it up later; it's a powerful reminder of the activists who fought to get those of us with health conditions these very protections.[2]

Of course, law does not automatically equal justice. Discrimination still happens every day in the workplace—often subtly, sometimes blatantly. We still have a long way to go in terms of equal opportunity and workplace understanding.

A few basics regarding the ADA:

- The ADA applies to employers with fifteen or more employees.
- Smaller businesses may still fall under state or local protection, although they may be exempt from certain federal ADA requirements.
- Even businesses with fewer than fifteen employees may be required to follow certain ADA provisions if they qualify as "public accommodations," such as a shop or a restaurant.
- If you're thinking, Wow, Marisa, this is a lot of legal language and I'm reading this on two hours of sleep, hang in there. I promise I'm keeping this as simple as possible.

Here's the part you need most:

You do not have to ask for an accommodation from an employer at the time of hiring unless you need it to pass the hiring test or you need an accommodation as soon as you begin working. If you're diagnosed months or years into the job, you still have the right to request what you need.

If you want to take a much deeper dive into your rights under the ADA, I'd urge you to start with the Job Accommodation Network website, which provides a plethora of information.[3]

### *What Does a Reasonable Accommodation Actually Look Like?*

What exactly is a reasonable accommodation, how do you request one, and what recourse is available if you are denied? A reasonable accommodation is simply a change that helps you do your job safely and effectively without creating major difficulty or cost for your employer. Vague, yes, I know. Let's break it down with some examples:

- **Flexible/Modified Schedules:** Ideal for those who need to receive a medical procedure or IV treatments weekly or monthly at a clinic. Discuss catching up on work in the evening or on a weekend.
- **Ergonomic Workstations and Equipment:** Perfect for people with arthritic conditions and/or mobility devices such as wheelchairs, those who need stand-up work desks, etc.
- **Office Desk/Space Moves:** I've had friends with conditions such as Crohn's and colitis have their office space or desk moved closer to restroom facilities. Other friends who use walkers or wheelchairs have asked for workspaces or offices to be close to the elevator and parking areas.
- **Lighting Requests:** For those of us with conditions like lupus and psoriasis, fluorescent lightbulbs can trigger flareups and

symptoms such as rashes, fever, sores and fatigue.[4] Ask for low UV-ray emitting lightbulb options as an accommodation.

Possibilities abound as accommodation options can be creative, highly individualized, and also negotiated in an interactive, collaborative process between the employee and the employer.

### *How to Request an Accommodation (Professionally and Powerfully, of Course)*

If you are interested in making a reasonable accommodation request, begin with a written document to your employer and/or HR supervisor that specifically describes the limitation—you do not need to give them a diatribe about your diagnosis. Explain the accommodation you need and how it will help you perform the *essential functions* of the job. If your employer asks for "proof of need," you can get a simple doctor's note outlining functional limitations. Remember, you are not required to give them a fully detailed medical history, ever.

### *If You Get Denied or Pushback*

Now, let's say you do everything required of you as an employee in terms of requesting a reasonable accommodation, and you get pushback. First, and this part is crucial: *Document. Every. Single. Thing.* Every conversation, email, request, response, and moment that feels even slightly discriminatory. Legally, you need to know that any employer who refuses to engage in the interactive process mentioned above, denies a reasonable accommodation without offering alternatives, fires or disciplines you after you disclose a need, or even penalizes you because of flare or medical-procedure related absences, can all be in violation of the ADA.

It's important to take ADA violations seriously and act swiftly. You can escalate to HR, but if things do not improve, or in more extreme cases, you can reach out to The Equal Employment Opportunity Commission, known as the EEOC. This organization handles all ADA-related issues; filing a claim is free and can lead to mediation between you and the employer, investigation, or even legal action taken against the employer. Remember: You deserve a workplace that supports your humanity, not one that punishes your biology.

### *Navigating Workplace Culture Amidst Illness*

While accommodations in and of themselves can feel tricky, navigating workplace culture with a chronic illness is a whole other story. It can feel like you were dropped into a foreign land when entering a workplace ecosystem and having a diagnosis in tow. For starters, most workplaces aren't built with chronic illness or disability in mind; they're built for "the healthies," the dependable 9–5 energy machines who don't know what it's like to not feel restored in any way after a weekend in bed.

Perhaps when you walk into the breakroom at your employer, coworkers are bragging about running marathons, being out late at a fun event, or jetting off to quick getaways, while you're thinking, *Whoa, I'm still recovering from last Tuesday's grocery run.* And if your illness is invisible, and you don't present like you just rolled out of a trash can, watch out: You will likely be met with bias immediately, because apparently looking "great" qualifies as the final say on your overall health.

If you currently find yourself in this workplace scenario, you might be wrestling with this common question: How much do I share and how much do I hold tight to my chest? Perhaps you have people within your immediate work environment that don't have the kindest hearts, people who have commented about how much time "you seem to take off," or mutter that your accommodation is unfair or is preferential treatment. How do we handle the emotional and psychological side of all this while just trying to do our jobs and not completely fall apart?

There's a lot to say; I'll try to keep it short-ish and only mildly spicy. Sorry, this topic really gets my gears in motion.

We spend a large portion of our life working and being surrounded by a variety of personalities. Navigating personality types is an art, in my opinion, even if you are doing it with a fully functioning immune system. For those of us who aren't, it requires even more creativity, decision-making, and boundary setting. First things first: *You are not legally required to disclose your illness to anyone at work* except HR or your supervisor *if* you need an accommodation or schedule change. Even then, what you share is entirely your choice. A few clear, short sentences usually do the job.

Because here are the facts: You are *not* the chronic-illness spokesperson for your entire office. You do not need to re-educate Chad from Sales every other week or justify your accommodation to Karen in Finance who insists she also has immune issues because she had a rash once twelve years ago. Can we not, Karen?

That said, being judged, dismissed, or not believed hurts. It can feel like high-school Mean Girls, except the adults are older, louder, and somehow even less self-aware. Navigating this psychological landmine requires boundaries, reframing, and protecting your spirit like it's your full-time job.

Enter into the subtle art of not internalizing other people's bullsh . . . um, nonsense. It's a life skill, a superpower, and a sanity-saver.

When someone comments, "Wow, it must be nice to work from home," or "Leaving early again?" or you overhear watercooler gossip about your new chair . . . deep breaths, my friend. This is where the internal work comes in.

First a reminder: People's lack of understanding isn't your lack of truth. This goes for the workplace as well as the rest of your life. Colleagues won't be the only ones questioning the validity of your condition. People interpret what they can and can't see through their own limited lens. They're reacting from ignorance, not insight. And ignorance is not your responsibility to fix.

There are two ways to reframe this experience: Cognitive diffusion and internal boundaries. Cognitive diffusion teaches you to step back from a negative and/or painful thought. An example? When a thought like, *They think I'm faking to get special treatment,* comes into your mind, take some space from it. Literally. Picture yourself taking a step back from that thought and say to yourself, *I am having the thought that they think this—but it's just a thought, not a fact.* It creates distance and keeps their noise from becoming your reality. You know the truth. You know why you are asking for an accommodation or change in schedule. The goal with cognitive diffusion techniques is to create distance and see thoughts as merely words, not truths. Continuing to do this each time a painful thought comes up helps you learn how to create emotional distance, and serves as a reminder that other people's disbelief and skepticism is not your self-concept and reality.

Next, it's time to create some internal boundaries. There will always be times at work and in everyday life, where external boundaries aren't respected by people. It's in these times that our internal boundaries can ground us and protect our peace and energy.

Internal boundaries can sound like:

I can't control what they think about me or my condition but I can control how I respond to it.

This person's opinion of my health journey is none of my business.

Their misunderstanding of my health is not my emergency.

These little mental shields protect your energy from other people's projections.

### *For The Times You Do Need to Respond*

Sometimes the work environment gets a little . . . *crunchy.* In the moments you feel prompted to verbally respond, there are ways to be kind *and* firm without losing your dignity or burning the place down. When someone continues to disrespect boundaries at work, continues with underhanded comments, or continues to push for information, have some rehearsed phrases tailored to your comfortability in your back pocket, such as:

"I'm working with my medical team and HR to create a plan that keeps me at my best. Thanks for your concern." Translation: Confidence while shutting down nosey-energy.

"I have a medical condition that affects me in various ways, but HR/my supervisor and I have it handled." Translation: Move along, Brenda; this doesn't concern you.

"I appreciate your concern; everything is under control." Translation: Ending the conversation immediately while still being professional.

"Thanks for asking! I'm managing things well and keeping things private." Translation: Exudes warm-balanced energy while not inviting more questions.

"I know you are genuinely asking me because you care. And I appreciate that. I am okay but keeping the details to myself." Translation: Affirms their intent while holding a solid boundary.

"Let's just say my immune system likes to beat its own drum. But the details aren't on tour right now." Translation: Humor + boundary = chef's kiss.

Phrases like these keep your privacy intact without igniting unnecessary workplace drama, 'cause, let's be real: we have enough with our own immune system.

### *Worth Doesn't Shrink Post-Diagnosis*

Workplace culture is unique to each company and field. You will meet busybodies, gossipers, skeptics, and people who cannot fathom what invisible illness is like. The reminder we must give ourselves is this: We have the choice to not let toxic or judgy workplace culture erode our worth.

You are navigating life, relationships, and work with a body that is trying to go rogue on a daily basis. You are full of determination, grit, and strength—characteristics some people will never understand or possess. And at the end of the day, we do not need a colleague's applause to know the worth we carry within.

Being chronically ill doesn't make us any less professional or creative or brilliant or perfectly suited for a job. In fact, I believe the traits that are refined alongside a chronic illness, such as resilience and adaptability, creative problem solving, strategic planning, empathy, emotional intelligence, determination, persistence, advocating, and phew, I could go on and on . . . these traits are what we bring to the workplace table and they are invaluable. Hint: Put these traits on your resume the next time you need to make one. We don't need anyone's approval to validate our worth—we already carry it within us.

### *Out With the Old: When a New Path Needs to be Discovered*

Chronic illness doesn't just affect your physical body, it can bring your entire career to a screeching halt. If you can no longer continue in the job you trained for or you spent years in school preparing for a profession that your body can no longer sustain and you're staring into the unknown thinking—*What now?*—we need to chat.

We live in a society that ties self-worth to productivity and worships hustle culture like it's a religion. So when chronic illness removes career stability, along with the finances, routine, community, and sense of purpose that came with it, the emotional fallout is very real. It can feel like losing a piece of your identity and "purpose."

But here is a reframe I encourage you to boldly step into: This isn't just an ending; it is actually the beginning of an entirely new chapter. What you define as purpose, productivity, and work is allowed to evolve, and with a chronic illness, it *needs to evolve.*

Sometimes that evolution means not working for a season. Sometimes it means part-time work, applying for assistance during brutal seasons, or completely reinventing yourself with a new career that honors your body's reality. And yes . . . as terrifying as it feels, reinvention can also be exciting. Reinvention can be empowering. Reinvention can be the moment you step into something even better than what you left behind.

I've had countless seasons of reframing and reinvention over the past twenty years. For many of those early years, I was unable to work *at all.* It wasn't about finding a new career at that point; my only job was staying alive and obviously, brushing my teeth. I drained my savings, maxed out my credit cards on medical bills, and moved back home with my mother and grandmother. It was not glamorous. It was not in my "life plan." But having that temporary cocoon, as financially messy as it was, allowed me to stabilize, identify my triggers, explore treatments, and slowly rebuild. Inch by inch, I regained tiny slices of normal life as months moved into years. I didn't need a nurse as often. Eventually, I could leave the house and partake in outings without ending up hospitalized. And eventually, I felt that little spark again, the spark that said, *Okay. Maybe I can rebuild a life. Maybe I'm finally ready to reinvent myself.*

During those first few years post-diagnosis, I could not return to nursing; lifting patients, long shifts, and germ exposure while on a boatload of immunosuppressants? Absolutely was not happening. And the grief of that situation was one of the hardest mourning periods for me to wade through. Letting go of a career you worked endlessly for is a profound mourning process. But when I finally reached the point of, *Okay, I may not be able to do nursing anymore, but I still have passion, skills, and abilities to help people in other ways,* something unlocked.

It was then that the magic happened.

A diagnosis can stop you from performing certain tasks for a season, but it doesn't strip you of your strengths: your work ethic, creativity, compassion, communication, strategy, problem-solving, empathy, and grit. These don't disappear the moment a doctor pronounces a diagnosis. These traits and strengths transfer. They evolve. And they can be repurposed beautifully.

I began listing my passions: writing, art, research, wellness, storytelling, teaching, and helping people. Then I asked: *What roles align with these passions, and what can my body handle right now?* Twenty years ago, yes, the options were limited. Today, the landscape of illness-friendly work environments is bigger than ever: remote roles, flexible jobs, freelance and consulting opportunities, hybrid environments, and creative careers that let you work in ways that support your health instead of running it completely into the ground.

I know dozens of people thriving in careers they never would have pursued if chronic illness hadn't nudged them onto a different path. If transitioning out of your current job feels terrifying, I want to encourage you: Something beautiful can be ahead. You are not trapped. You are not finished. You are simply being rerouted.

Let me help you build that new map.

## A Fun, Creative Framework for Your New Career Path

When you are in the mindset and energy space to do a quick exercise, grab a notebook or open up a blank Word document because things are about to get exciting. We are going to work together and you are going to design work around your life, not the other way around.

### *Step 1. Reflection: What Lights You Up vs. What Drains You?*

Ask yourself the following questions and jot your answers down somewhere for safe-keeping:

- ***What Energizes Me?*** These are tasks you naturally fall into and can completely lose track of time. It can be anything from writing, painting, organizing, designing, creating content, coaching, researching, analyzing data, speaking to people about a topic you are obsessed with, etc. What you will notice with the activities that energize you is this: They don't bulldoze your nervous and immune system; they actually support it by releasing feel-good chemicals.

- ***What Drains Me?*** Next, think about the tasks or roles that cause an immediate internal scream, fatigue, pain, tension, brain fog, or complete mental/physical exhaustion. This list is critical because whatever path you decide to take in your future career endeavor, it should contain as few of these tasks as possible. Now, it may be impossible to eliminate all of them but we don't want these tasks to run the bulk of your "job."

This is the first part of the trail toward a career map that works alongside your body, not against it every day.

### *Step 2. Your Ideal Workday and Environment*

Next, we are going to extract some helpful data by visualizing your current season of health:

- What time of day does your energy peak?
- What time of day does your energy crash?
- What sensory needs do you need to take into account such as light, temperature, noise, mobility factors, etc.?
- How mobile are you on a scale of 1–10 on your baseline "decent" days? How about on your flare days? Be honest with yourself, here!
- How difficult is it for you to concentrate if you have a day where brain fog is a factor?
- Do you like to work independently or within a team setting?
- How realistic is a job out of the home or is remote/hybrid an absolute must?
- Are there any environments you would like to avoid? (For me it's hospitals and medical settings because of the germs).

These answers help you form the branches of the path of your future career—even if your work is officially completely from the couch!

### *Step 3. The Feelings You Desire in Your Next Career*

You might be wondering why this even matters, but it does. Your emotional and mental health have a direct impact on your physical health. And with a chronic illness, we need as many feel-good chemicals coursing through our body as we can get.

Ask yourself and jot down the answers to:

- Do I desire more flexibility?
- Do I want a more creative role?
- What level of leadership am I interested in? Do I want to be in charge of a team or have less pressure and only be in charge of myself?
- What do I consider a sense of contribution to the world in terms of using my gifts and strengths?
- Is a slower pace more important to me in this season?
- How do I feel about a role that is more aligned with the person I have become during this season of my life?

The ultimate goal is to not just find a job but to build a career and lifestyle that fits into our daily health speed-bumps.

### *Step 4. Track Your "Capacity Curve"*

In this part of the exercise, you will want to take your "capacity curve" into consideration, meaning how your body's bandwidth fluctuates from day to day. To determine your unique capacity curve, track the following for the next seven to fourteen days:

- When are your energy high and low points each day?
- Determine how much you can get done on a "normal baseline" day, such as how many hours per day you can concentrate on tasks, how many naps you need, how many good "workable hours" hours in the day you typically have where your energy is stable.
- Next, determine the same for a "flare day"—you may not be able to do anything on these days except sit in bed and breathe. This is perfectly acceptable, just be honest with yourself and make note of it.
- Track your mobility over the seven to fourteen days: how many breaks did you need, did you nap, are you able to lift items, run errands easily or did you need assistance and/or a mobility device?
- Think about your sensory needs, such as noise, light, temperature, etc. over this seven-to-fourteen-day period and determine what you can and cannot tolerate.

Why do we want to track all of this information for a good week or two? Because the difference between a sustainable career and one that destroys your physical and mental health is knowing what you can *realistically do* on both good days and terrible ones.

Think of these exercises as discovering your "user manual." Is your future career being a cashier or bank teller for forty hours a week on your feet, working out of the home, and engaging with large amounts of people? Maybe that is completely out of the question. But can it be a remote marketing assistant for twenty hours a week with flexible deadlines? That might be a thousand times more realistic.

### *Step 5. Testing Potential Ideas Before Committing*

If there is anything I can share with you about my wild and all-over-the-map job endeavors post diagnosis, it is this: if you have a way to test a potential career first, before diving in headfirst only to learn it puts you into a flare/hospital two weeks later, do it!

Here are a few ideas for safely test-driving your career ideas:

- **Interview someone in the field.** Ask them to share what an average day is, in addition to what they love and don't love about their career? A sixty-minute Zoom conversation can save you months of guesswork, schooling you may not need to invest in, and potentially worsening of symptoms.
- **Try a low-cost or free online class.** There are so many low-pressure ways to explore a potential new skill which could lead to a new career. Skillshare, Coursera, YouTube, and many universities online offer free to low-cost videos or courses on endless subject matters.
- **Volunteer a few hours a week.** If possible, immerse yourself in the environment and allow your body *to tell you* if the work is truly a sustainable choice.
- **Engage in micro-gigs or projects.** Create profiles or stores on sites like Etsy, Upwork, Fiverr, Faire and more to showcase your skills, creations, art, etc. and gauge the interest over time.
- **Audit your energy while doing any of the above.** Whatever test-drive option you try, ask yourself the following as you engage: Did this energize me? Did it cause symptoms? Did I need a recovery period after? Do I believe I could do this consistently?

By testing ideas first, you are protecting your body, your future and your hope.

### *Step 6. Decide if Illness Plays a Role in Your New Career*

Some of us have reshaped our pain into our new career "purpose" (this book is just one example). Perhaps this interests you—and it's also okay if it doesn't. You absolutely do not have to build a career around your diagnosis if that is "not your cup of tea." But for some people, their lived experience pre- and post-diagnosis becomes a powerful and major part of their future work.

If the idea of this interests you, here are some ways one's illness story can integrate into a career:

- Writing blogs, content, books, articles.
- Advocating through speaking, mentoring, collaborating with government officials, raising awareness through social media, etc.
- Turning emotion into creative expression through art, song, poetry, and dance.
- Coaching and guiding others through their own health journeys or life transitions.
- Entrepreneurship by creating and designing products, techs, fashion, services, or resources that weren't available to you when you needed them most.
- Joining or founding a nonprofit organization (I did this by founding LupusChick).

Those who intertwine their story into their future career path may find the combination empowering and healing on many levels. But again, this is optional. Your illness story can also just be one piece of the structure without becoming the entire home.

Are your wheels spinning yet? Perhaps you are wondering what some of the most popular chronic-illness-friendly career choices are? I asked my community and here were some of the top answers:

- Graphic design, photo editing, illustration
- Social media management and marketing, digital content creation
- Writing, editing, and proofreading
- Bookkeeping, transcription, data entry
- Web design, coding, UX design
- Customer support, virtual assistant
- Remote administrative work
- Research, data analyst, grant writing
- Creative roles and patient advocacy/illness-related careers
- Coaching or consulting in your expertise areas
- Freelance and/or entrepreneurial ventures built around your stamina and interests

After forging an entirely new career for myself, one that aligned with my needs, passions, and my body, I fully believe you can and will find your perfect fit too. And just keep in mind, your "perfect" new career may evolve over time as you get to know your body more intimately. You will discover work that feeds your spirit, respects your body, and supports you financially.

Your new post-diagnosis superpower? You no longer have to squeeze yourself into the world's 9–5 box. You get to build your own.

## When Working Is *Not* a Viable Option

I'm not a psychic but . . . who knows, maybe somewhere down the road you'll launch your own business, step on a stage to speak, create art, or move into a career you never saw coming. But right now? Maybe you are simply trying to just survive the sheer chaos you've been dropped into, and actively working in this very season is not possible. At all. Not even for an hour a week. Been there. And it feels terrible, emotionally, physically, and also financially.

If that's where you are, imagine me sitting across from you, looking directly into your tired, overwhelmed eyes and saying:

"I know this is terrifying. I know it feels lonely. And I know you're exhausted from fighting battles most people can't see. But this moment is not your forever. This is a 'just right now.'"

If your body is in full revolt and work is off the table, you may need to apply for assistance in terms of unemployment, Medicaid, Social Security disability, and other support programs in your area. And yes, I am aware that even just thinking about applying can poke at your pride. Many of us spent years being the one who "figures everything out," so admitting we need help can feel like emotional whiplash. Add paperwork, doctor's notes, endless doctor's visits and tests, medical records, forms that read like ancient scripture, and brain fog? It's a lot.

But hear me clearly: These programs exist because even the strongest, most resilient people need a life raft sometimes. They can help cover the cost of medications you cannot live without. They can keep the lights on and food in the refrigerator. They can buy you time to stabilize, to rest, to rebuild. They are a bridge, not a definition of your worth.

If you're cringing while reading this but you're also choosing between buying medication or groceries, here's a reframe to help soothe the discomfort: *I'm applying for help so I can survive this season well enough to make it to my next one.*

### *Where to Find Help and What to Expect*

Reaching out for help can happen in a variety of ways. In addition to Medicaid and Social Security Disability (SSDI and SSI), many states and counties have additional assistance programs. Two helpful starting places:

**Findhelp.org**—enter your ZIP code and access countless local resources for food, housing, emergency funds, transportation, treatment support, and more.
**Healthcare.gov**—to explore Medicaid and low-cost health coverage options in your state.

Medicaid is a joint federal and state program that can help cover essential medical, hospital, and long-term care services in addition to prescription drugs. You can apply for Medicaid online at your state's Medicaid website or through Healthcare.gov. In addition, SSDI and SSI (through the Social Security Administration, SSA) are federal disability programs that can help chronically ill/disabled persons with limited income and resources.

Both are long, often frustrating processes, especially for people living with chronic illnesses that don't have clear imaging or one "classic" diagnostic test.

Here's what you should know before moving forward with either of the programs through SSA:

- **Documentation is everything.** SSDI looks at *functional limitations*, not just your diagnosis. Keep symptoms diaries, your medical records, and any letters written by doctors, treatment history, lab results, functional assessments, and any notes or journals detailing how the illness affects your daily life and activities of daily living—see how often this comes up?

With these types of federal assistance programs, patterns matter. Consistency matters. Specificity matters.

- **Expect denials.** And remember, it is not personal; it's how the system is designed. In fact, up to 70 percent of first applications are denied. But many are overturned during appeals (some data shows up to 50 percent).[5] So don't let the first "no" send you into a shame spiral and stop you from appealing.
- **Hiring a disability lawyer can help and costs nothing upfront.** Disability lawyers only get paid if you get approval and only from a small portion of your back pay. So, for zero money out of pocket, let them do a lot of the heavy lifting like helping gather evidence, strengthen your case, prepare testimony, and fight on your behalf.
- **The SSA timeline will test every nerve you have left. Every one, I promise.** This process can take months or years and may impact you financially and emotionally. I guarantee there will be a moment when you want to throw papers up in the air and scream. But you are not weak for applying or needing help. You are not easily swayed. KEEP GOING FORWARD. You are choosing survival and safety until you're able to move into your next chapter.

And please, for the love of your nervous system, don't let the SSA approval rollercoaster beat you down. Appeals can be incredibly successful. Let your lawyer fight the fight. Your job is to heal and love on your body that is struggling right now.

## It's a Work Wrap

You and I have traveled a long road just now regarding career and chronic illness—wading through grief, our rights, workplace culture, advocacy, reinvention, and the brutally tender reality of needing to ask for help when working is out of the question. If those closest around you haven't said this to you lately, let me be the one: You are doing your best. You are working with a hurting body that is in desperate need of rest and healing all while being trapped in a society that is literally obsessed with hustle culture and speed.

There's no sugar coating it: Your career path from this moment forward will look different, but it can hold creativity, purpose, flexibility and possibility. As you navigate this rocky road, remember you haven't failed or fallen behind, even when it feels like others are gaining momentum. You are building a career path that supports and sustains what you and your body need in this very season. Your brilliance, experience, and countless character strengths aren't going anywhere. Not only are you still in the game, I think you are actually ahead of the game—one where you play smarter, gentler and on your own terms.

## CHAPTER 8

# MEDICAL PTSD, TRAUMA, AND OTHER PARTY CRASHERS

In early 2025, I launched a podcast with my "spoonie" sidekick, Britt, through LupusChick called *I'd Like to Unsubscribe.* And yes, I know, another podcast. Go, go Gadget eyeroll. But stay with me for a minute. While there are plenty of podcasts out there speaking about mental health and psychology, what I couldn't find much of—and what I felt so many of us were starving for—are these topics solely investigated through the lens of chronic illness. Millions upon millions of us are white-knuckling our way through the mental health rollercoaster that comes with being diagnosed with a lifelong condition. So why aren't we openly discussing the mental pressure that comes along with existing in a sick body?

This topic is anything but new for me. I started trying to have this exact conversation over twenty years ago, when I took my first job as a health journalist. I wrote an article that tried to explain the mental chaos lupus had introduced into my life, using the only metaphor that made sense at the time: a backpack. And my message to the reader was this: Imagine wearing a backpack filled with jagged rocks all day, every day. In my mind, each rock was labeled with some part of the "mental load" of chronic illness: appointments to remember, medications to take on schedule, calculating how much energy is left in your tank, deciding what tasks get sacrificed today, showing up for family and friends, being present for your partner, managing guilt, fear, chronic pain, fatigue, financial strain, and grieving the hobbies you no longer have energy for.

*Phew.* And that wasn't even half of it. . . .

For so long, it felt like no one could even fathom what was inside that backpack; perhaps they thought it contained just a notebook or some granola bars. They couldn't see the sharp edges, the heaviness, the way it pressed into my chest and made it hard to breathe. And because no one else seemed to notice, I convinced myself I shouldn't mention it either. This was my life now. My cross to bear. So, I silenced my voice, not sharing the anxiety and fear and the relentless, exhausting rumination about how I was going to survive one more day under the weight of it all.

I wish I could tell you I got a break from the heaviness once I closed my eyes at night, but instead, sleep became yet another battleground. There was no peace at the end of the day as I always hoped. Instead, I started having vivid nightmares; my body reenacting every trauma, every procedure, every moment of uncertainty I'd shoved down during the day. My nervous system was staging a full-blown protest instead of relaxing and repairing itself in those late-night hours.

And then, one day out of nowhere, the metaphorical pot finally boiled over.

I had my first panic attack.

And let me tell you: It scared the absolute s*&% out of me.

I was driving one afternoon and my chest suddenly squeezed. At first, I assumed my asthma was staging a rare mutiny, perhaps triggered by springtime allergens in the South Florida air—a common occurrence around that time of year. But within seconds I knew something else was happening. This felt wildly different. My throat felt like invisible hands were closing around it and as I drove with one hand, the other was frantically massaging the sides of my neck. Taking a full, deep breath became impossible. And soon enough, my body started trembling and my teeth chattered.

I swerved into a patch of grass near the Fort Lauderdale airport, flung my door open, and fell to my knees. I dug both hands deep into the crunchy grass and warm dirt as if it was the only thing tethering me to earth. And then I vomited. When the shaking finally subsided, I crawled back into the car, curled into the fetal position and cried until my ribs hurt. I stayed like that for hours, too terrified to move, pleading with God to please allow whatever that was to never happen again.

I truly thought it was a one-off. A fluke. A reaction to something I ate. Or just a weird moment in a challenging year.

It wasn't.

Instead, it was the beginning of a multi-year chapter of my life that included crippling panic attacks that left me unable to drive or even get inside of a car most days, for almost a year. In what felt like the snap of a finger, my independence evaporated. My world, already shrunken so much by illness, contracted even further. It felt like a cruel cosmic joke. *What else could possibly be taken from me?* I wondered.

"Marisa, have you ever heard of the phrase Medical PTSD?" my new therapist asked me after that incident. I hadn't; remember, it was still basically the dark ages tech-wise (circa 2005-ish). There were no reels, no carousels, no Tik-Tok therapists or coaches breaking down the framework of Medical PTSD in sixty seconds with soothing music in the background. No community conversations about medical trauma, and definitely no one validating what I was experiencing or why it wasn't surprising given everything I had been through.

So, when he said those words and explained it all, everything began to make sense. Of course the panic attacks finally erupted. Of course my body was sounding alarms in any way it possibly could to get my attention. I had been lugging around major, unprocessed medical trauma every single day, stuffed deep down into that heavy backpack. Never putting it down; never taking a day off.

If you aren't familiar with my story, hold on to your seatbelt. My official lupus diagnosis came shortly after I was run over by a pick-up-truck while crossing a street one night in Fort Lauderdale. Yes, you read that right. Literally run over as a pedestrian, by a drunk driver. I sustained horrific injuries and spent nearly a year in the hospital and rehab rebuilding myself piece by piece. And just when I thought I was reaching the finish line of recovery from one of the most horrific events of my life, I got handed a fun new diagnosis to figure out. Not too long after that bombshell, I had a small stroke and, coupled with the injuries from the truck, I was sent off to rehabilitation to learn how to walk again.

And remember: Before anyone muttered the word *lupus* to me, I had already spent fifteen years being dismissed, doubted, or told "It's just your allergies." Fifteen years of being sick and unheard. Even after the diagnosis, some doctors still didn't believe me. I was either "too young," or I "looked fine."

And while we are on the topic of good ol' trauma (this time with a sprinkle of gaslighting too), there was one ER visit I'll never forget. I was experiencing my first ever pulmonary embolism from a blood clot that had apparently traveled from my leg and decided to lodge itself in an artery in my lung. My oxygen saturation was at eighty percent. I was gasping like a fish on a dock, my airway feeling about as wide open as a coffee stirrer straw. The ER doctor glanced at my chart, glanced at my face, and said, "You probably just need to get out in the Florida sun more." The audacity!

Sir.

My guy.

I was *actively dying*, not vitamin D deficient.

What I'd love to say to that man, and yes, he should've been fired, but that's another story for another book.

My point is this: If any of this feels eerily familiar—if you are reading these words and thinking, *Oh, that's me*, and you've never heard of Medical PTSD or your doctor never mentioned it after your diagnosis or traumatic medical experience, please hear me: Medical PTSD is real trauma response. Not imagined. Not you being "dramatic."

It happens when the nervous system becomes so completely overwhelmed by medical experiences that it can no longer distinguish past danger from present safety. Your body stays stuck in survival mode: panic, fear, hypervigilance, and dread. And your body has learned, through lived experience, that the places you were told could heal you were also the places that hurt you.

So, when someone casually says in the midst of your panic and fear to an upcoming procedure or unexpected ER visit, "Oh, no one likes going to the hospital. Just relax, you'll be fine," it's almost laughable. *Relaxing* literally does not translate in the brain when you are experiencing Medical PTSD. *Relaxing* doesn't register with your nervous system when it feels like you are walking back into the lion's den and your brain is screaming: "I've been here before and it didn't go well. Abort! Abort!"

This isn't thinking negatively or you being reluctant to do something. This is an actual trauma response where your brain correlates things like hospitals, procedures, medical emergencies and symptoms directly to danger, potentially life-threatening, and terrifying. And so, your nervous system never quite calms down, but instead feels like it needs to stay on high alert in order to protect you. All the time. At all costs. Even when the threat has passed.

Events and/or triggers that fall under the Medical PTSD umbrella can look like: years of being misdiagnosed and dismissed; a painful or invasive procedure; a brutal recovery; a near-death emergency; being spoken to with cruelty and skepticism in the midst of a medical crisis; a critical flare that required rapid, life-saving care; or the slow, devastating loss of autonomy as your health declines.

It could also be processing that painful collision between the story society tells us— *hospitals are safe and doctors help you get better*—and what you have actually lived through. And it's not that you don't want to believe that story the world teaches. You *try* to believe it. But your nervous system remembers every moment of terror and heartbreak. And at the end of the day, our internal alarm system doesn't give a damn about societal narratives. It cares about surviving.

So, is it any wonder the body and mind brace for impact when we step into that follow-up visit or a medical setting?

And because we are dealing with chronic illness—the forever subscription we never signed up for—these scary health moments rarely come as a single episode in our life. They often stack on top of each other as the years go by: a worrisome procedure here, a life-changing diagnosis there, toss in a terrifying allergic reaction you never saw coming. Layer after layer after layer. Until one day the stack becomes too heavy for any human to shoulder, and something cracks.

And just like that, the alarm bells go off.

So, what's actually happening in the body when Medical PTSD rears its head? And why does your whole system go DEFCON 1 at the sight of a tourniquet or hospital gown? Whether it's one traumatic event or ten or, let's be honest, two hundred, the underlying biology is the same: Medical PTSD alters how the brain functions and sometimes also alters the structure and size of certain brain regions. Over time, it rewires the nervous system into a permanent state of "I'm-not-letting-my-guard-down-for-a-second" survival mode.

And here's the thing: Your body is truly a magnificent creation even though we don't always feel this way. It is always working hard to protect you. *Always*. It doesn't take a day off. But what happens when that protection mode doesn't take a moment off, even in situations where you are absolutely safe? When the guard dog inside your brain's alarm control center continues to bark long after the threat (or UPS guy) is gone? This is where the reality of living with Medical PTSD becomes exhausting.

Medically speaking, several parts of the brain are involved with Medical PTSD, but three major players take center stage: **the amygdala, the prefrontal cortex, and the hippocampus.**[1] If you can't remember high school biology (other than the frog dissection), here's your crash course—minus the pop quiz.

### *The Amygdala: The Body's Internal Alarm System (like ADT without the monthly fee)*

Think of the amygdala as the smoke detector of your brain. Its job is to scan for danger and, if it senses even a whiff of threat, slam its hand on the panic button. With PTSD, the amygdala becomes *over*-reactive. So, in time, it basically becomes a toddler with a bullhorn: loud, dramatic, and completely uninterested in logic and what is actually happening.

So even in those moments when you are fully safe, say sitting in your cozy bed, scrolling on Insta, reminding yourself this is "just a checkup," your amygdala may be flipping the body's stress-response switch like you're being chased by Michael Myers.

### The Prefrontal Cortex: The Voice of Reason (Now silenced)

The prefrontal cortex is the rational part of your brain: Imagine it as the mature adult in the room, the calm grandmother that says, "Let's sit down, honey, and think this through." It is responsible for a lot: regulating our emotions, thinking rationally, and making decisions. The issue is, when Medical PTSD occurs, it becomes impaired, can even change in size, and exhibits reduced activity.

Once impaired, it becomes really difficult for the brain to send signals to the amygdala that there truly is no danger lurking. It gets completely drowned out by the amygdala's all-caps screaming. This is why you can *know* you're safe and still feel like your body is preparing for battle.

Logic never wins when biology is in survival mode.

### The Hippocampus: The Memory Keeper (Now confused)

Then there is the hippocampus, the part of the brain that processes and organizes all of our memories, helping us distinguish the past from present. When trauma and Medical PTSD come along, the hippocampus becomes less responsive and defunct, and even physically smaller in some cases, making scary events from our past feel as if they are happening right now. Now disrupted, your brain can't store memories correctly, so a particular smell, a tone in voice, a familiar room can pull you back into a terrifying moment from your past, even though you are currently not in danger.

Even though it is struggling, I promise you your brain isn't intentionally trying to torture you; it believes it is truly protecting you. This is the biological blueprint of Medical PTSD. It's not us having nothing better to do with our time so we overreact or become dramatic. It's our defunct nervous system doing the best it can to keep us alive but using outdated data from a past moment when danger was present.

And when all of these brain regions stop operating the way they're meant to, the delicate balance between our sympathetic nervous system (the one that rings the alarm) and our parasympathetic nervous system (the one that soothes and steadies us) gets completely turned on its head.

Is it any wonder the phrase, "You just need to calm down already and take a deep breath" muttered from your Aunt Karen across the dinner table does not work? Never in the history of telling someone with PTSD to "calm down" has anyone ever actually calmed the hell down.

And I say all of this to you because if your body and brain are currently in the throes of Medical PTSD, I know how terrifying, how disorienting, and how utterly overwhelming it can feel. Before that therapist ever spoke the words *Medical PTSD* to me, long before I understood the science behind what was functionally and structurally happening inside my brain, I spent many years beating myself up.

The lectures I gave myself were endless: Why can't you just think rationally about this?

Why are you freaking out again, Marisa? Get it together, girl!

I genuinely believed I could cheerlead my way out of biology that was working against me. But I have a spoiler for you: You will never be able to drill sergeant or pep-talk your way out of a nervous system in crisis.

If you take away only one thing from this book, please let it be this: If you are in the wilderness season of Medical PTSD right now, shower yourself with grace, patience, and tenderness. Offer yourself the same compassion you have given freely to others. Working through Medical PTSD, no matter which path you take (and we'll talk through those shortly), is not a 24-hour turnaround. Or a week turnaround. It's intentional work. Gentle work. Sometimes grueling work. And you deserve love, support, and tenderness as you navigate and process it all.

And . . . as you're working through it, in those moments when partners or family or friends don't understand why you "can't just talk yourself out of it," you have numerous options. You can educate them kindly, you can set boundaries firmly, or you can (politely or not—your prerogative) serve up one of the following responses:

### *If You Want to Provide a Biological Breakdown*

"My brain is firing survival signals from past, terrifying experiences. That's why I can't 'snap out' of panic. My body isn't being dramatic; it's actually trying to protect me based on trauma. Therapy is helping me rewire this, but it doesn't happen overnight."

### *Asking Them to Stop in a Firm but Loving Way*

"When you tell me I just need to calm down or stop thinking negatively, it actually makes me feel worse, like I am failing at something

I can't biologically control. What I need right now is understanding and love, and someone who will be there for me as I work through this."

### *The Kind, "No-filter" Reality Check*

"Trust me, if I could rationalize my way out of this, I would have done it a long time ago. But now I understand biologically what I am processing is stored trauma; it has nothing to do with me being weak or negative. I could use some understanding and love as I work with my coach/therapist on retraining my nervous system."

### *Offer The Heart + Science Explanation*

"I'm working through Medical PTSD which is tied to changes in the brain and the body's fight or flight response. Even when I am technically safe, my brain believes I'm in immediate danger. I wish I could just talk myself out of what is biologically happening, but healing trauma requires I do nervous system retraining. Your support while I work through this means everything."

Though Medical PTSD can feel both challenging and frightening, you'll notice a common thread woven in those sample responses above: *The nervous system can be retrained.* Yes, trauma can imprint itself on the brain and create negative neuroplastic changes, but here's the part that still feels like a tiny miracle to me: Those changes do not have to be permanent.

We can harness neuroplasticity, the brain's incredible ability to adapt, change, and reorganize itself for our healing. Through a variety of different practices and therapies that encourage "positive" neuroplastic shifts, we can create new neural pathways and gradually regain a sense of control, steadiness, and well-being. The key to working through Medical PTSD is consistency. Repetition. Intention. Showing up again and again for whichever practice or therapy you choose, even on the days you feel like a melted candle that's headed straight for the trash can. Healing happens in small, steady rewires, not overnight transformations.

There are a wide variety of practices and evidence-based strategies you can explore when you are ready. Below is a high-level overview of each to help you guide your decision.

If you naturally gravitate toward more evidence-based psychotherapy practices, you might want to consider:

**Eye Movement Desensitization and Reprocessing (EMDR)**

EMDR is a trauma-focused therapy that many people (myself included) find incredibly helpful when medical trauma has imprinted itself on the nervous system. Simply put, EMDR helps the brain *reprocess* traumatic memories so they don't carry the same emotional punch or send your body into shutdown, panic, or full-body implosion mode every time something reminds you of the original event.

This therapy uses bilateral stimulation, often guided eye movements, tapping, or tones, to engage both hemispheres of the brain while you revisit aspects of the memory in a safe, regulated environment. And let's be crystal clear about this therapy choice: EMDR does not erase the memory. It's not brain bleaching. Instead, it helps your brain *re-file* the memory, moving it from the disorganized file drawer that is labeled "EMERGENCY" into one that your brain can process without hitting the panic button.

Over time, the emotional intensity you experience attached to the memory begins to soften. The physical reactivity decreases. And, if and when a trigger pops up later, your nervous system no longer treats it like the beginning of a medical thriller. Many people with Medical PTSD find EMDR especially effective because it works directly with the parts of the brain that store trauma. No more forcing yourself to "logic" your way out of something your body encoded as danger.

***Who might find EMDR helpful?***

- People who have vivid, intense flashbacks or body memories
- People who feel traditional talk therapy hasn't moved the needle
- People who begin to spiral inside certain medical environments
- People who experience their body reacting before the brain even knows why

EMDR can be a powerful reset button for a nervous system that has forgotten how to stand down.

**Cognitive Processing Therapy (CPT)**

CPT is another evidence-based approach worth exploring; its goal is to help someone identify and challenge the "unhelpful beliefs" known as *stuck points* that occur after a traumatic event and typically hinder one's recovery. These are the sneaky thoughts, deeply rooted in fear, that shape how you see your body, your safety, the medical system, and yourself.

You might be wondering, *what does a stuck point sound like in my mind?* Think of stuck points as the brain's unhelpful post-trauma narrators. They might sound similar to:

- **Self-blame:** "I should've known better."

- **Fear-based assumptions:** "Doctors will *never* believe me when I'm sick."
- **Hopelessness:** "I'll never be safe in my body."
- Or having rigid rules about trust, control, or vulnerability.

CPT's various exercises help you trace these beliefs back to where they started, examine the evidence *and truth* behind them (spoiler: You'll be surprised how many beliefs crumble under real scrutiny), and gently replace them with perspectives that are more accurate, compassionate and balanced.

Using guided exercises and cognitive restructuring, CPT gives your brain the opportunity to revisit the memory on a neutral ground, not in that house of horrors your trauma built. And research shows, over time, this therapy can significantly reduce emotional reactivity, anxiety, and panic responses in medical settings. *I think almost everyone reading this book will take that, right?!*

***So who can truly benefit from CPT?***

- If your trauma changed the way you see yourself or the world
- If you carry shame or self-blame about past medical experiences
- If your fear feels cognitive more than physiological
- If you desire to try a structured, thought-focused approach

CPT is particularly powerful for those of us who feel "stuck" in the stories left behind by trauma.

**Other Psychotherapies to Consider**

If EMDR or CPT don't feel like your path, there are additional evidence-based options to consider as you navigate your healing. These include Narrative Exposure Therapy, which helps someone build a more coherent narrative of *all* life events, so memories that are traumatic lose their power and become just part of a larger story about you; and also, Prolonged Exposure Therapy, where you work with a professional to safely and gradually confront triggers that remind you of the trauma. In time, your brain rewires to understand this is not dangerous to me anymore.

### *Holistic, Body-Based Approaches*

Like me, you might find yourself drawn to more holistic therapies that don't just engage the mind, but the entire nervous system. The approaches below work beautifully alongside psychotherapy, or individually, especially if you're someone who feels emotions in your body before you ever find the right words for them. (Hi, it's me. I'm someone!)

### *Somatic Experiencing (SE)*

SE is built on the idea that trauma gets "stuck" in the nervous system when our natural survival impulses, good ol' fight-flight-or-freeze, were interrupted at the exact moment of trauma. And, for many of us with chronic illness, that disruption was inevitable.

Maybe you were immobilized on a hospital bed, hooked up to machines, unable to run, protest, or even speak up for yourself. SE helps you reclaim the inner authority and necessary instinctive completion that trauma interrupted.

This therapy guides you through full awareness of your body and allows you to have a safe place where you can finally resolve that response. It might involve breath work, micro-movements, gently shaking your body, vocalizations, and grounding/orienting exercises.

Through SE, the nervous system is reminded that the threat is now over, you have made it through, and you can finally relax. Think of it as a quiet unwinding of a tangled body, finally bringing the response your body needed to have initially to full completion.

The goal of SE is to remind the nervous system that the threat is now gone, you survived, and it's okay to stop scanning for danger.

SE is often a great fit if:

- You felt trapped, voiceless, or immobilized during the traumatic experience
- You are seeking a gentler, slow, non-retraumatizing modality
- Medical triggers spiral you into freeze, numb, or panic mode
- You feel disconnected or betrayed by your body and are ready to build a healthier relationship with it.

## Trauma-Informed Yoga

One of my favorite tools of the healing journey has been gentle, trauma-informed yoga. This practice can rebuild a trusting and safe relationship with the body, something I believe many of us lose after we experience a traumatic event; we no longer feel at home in our bodies, and it begins to feel more like a silo of chaos where unpredictable things can happen.

This type of yoga uses mindful, slow movements, gentle stretches, grounding postures, and breathwork that can help calm the fight or flight response. This yoga practice also engages the vagus nerve through humming and soft sounds, in addition to extended exhalations that help lessen anxiety and feelings of panic. There is no pressure to perform when partaking in trauma-informed yoga; you aren't engaging in this practice solely for fitness purposes. The goal is you reconnecting with your body in a compassionate way, a gentle whisper that says:

"My body and I are learning to trust each other again."

"My body is a place I can safely return to."

### *Who might love trauma-informed yoga?*

- Anyone seeking a compassionate and non-verbal practice
- Anyone who feels disconnected from his/her body
- Anyone looking for gentle, grounding modalities vs. intensity

### Additional mind-body therapies worth exploring?

You may feel more comfortable with neurofeedback, which uses real-time brainwave feedback that helps you retrain your nervous system to become more regulated; craniosacral therapy, which is hands-on and used to release tension and bring calm to an overstimulated nervous system. People who can most benefit from this therapy tend to physically carry trauma in their neck, jaw, and diaphragm; and last, but certainly not least, hypnotherapy, which can help you reframe existing subconscious beliefs rooted in fear and helplessness.

### *Psychedelic-Assisted Therapies*

Though I have not personally tried any of the following therapies, I feel I would be doing a disservice to you if these aren't mentioned. So much more research and trial completion has taken place in recent years and new treatment opportunities have become available when it comes to emerging therapies such as psilocybin, MDMA, and ketamine. While these options are not considered first-line treatments and must be administered in a clinic, they have shown promising results for complex trauma and medical PTSD. These therapies may help quiet down the brain's fear centers so you can revisit traumatic memories and work through the emotions without feeling like you are reliving the event in real time.

*Ayahuasca (A more nuanced option)*

Real talk: I am wildly intrigued and somewhat terrified of Ayahuasca, though I've never tried it (yet). It is appearing more often in trauma-healing conversations, though it is *not* considered a first line treatment nor is it medically supervised the way MDMA and psilocybin trials are. This traditional Amazonian plant medicine is believed to help people access blocked emotions, memories, and insights through altered states of consciousness. It is believed to work by reducing activity in the brain's "fear center," the amygdala we spoke of earlier, allowing participants to revisit trauma with less fear and greater perspective.

You'll find a divided camp on the topic of Ayahuasca and I would encourage ample research and conversations with past participants if you are considering taking part in a ceremony. Because here is the reality: Ayahuasca is not a gentle modality. The experience is said to be emotionally intense, physically demanding, and not safe for everyone (especially for people on certain medications). The healing potential of this option sits heavily on the knowledge of the facilitator, the safety of the environment, and your own mental and physical health.

When considering your path forward in healing from Medical PTSD, you may ultimately find that the best approach for you is weaving together a combination of both psychotherapy *and* holistic therapies—approaches that help you gently face the past while also creating present-moment safety, carving new neural pathways that softly whisper: "You're safe now. You made it. You can rest."

### *Mapping Out* Your *Journey*

Last, we can't discuss mapping out your healing journey without acknowledging co-occurring conditions that commonly show up like uninvited guests in the chronic illness community—particularly depression, anxiety, and chronic pain. A massive analysis of more than 375 studies consisting of 347,468 adults, completed by investigators at Johns Hopkins Medicine, found that as many as 40 percent of people living with chronic illness and pain experience "clinically significant depression and anxiety," with "women and younger adults" being the most at risk.[2]

All of this makes perfect sense when you zoom out and take in the full landscape: the life-shattering diagnosis that split time into *before* and *after*, the lifestyle changes, the medical trauma, the battles fought silently behind closed doors, and a body that suddenly works as well as dial-up internet during a bad thunderstorm. All of these things literally create the "perfect storm" for complete overwhelm to occur. Of course our mental health feels the aftershocks. Of course anxiety and depression slither in.

We don't live in a society designed to help navigate chronic illness. In fact, it's quite the opposite; we are told to smile, stay small, don't complain, and just "be happy you don't have it worse." And so we shove everything into the metaphorical backpacks I spoke of, strap them to our spines, and drag them through our lives—and we suffer. Sometimes for decades.

But that worn-out narrative of "just stay silent and be grateful"? We are moving beyond that now. Because the longer we sit in silence and just carry the trauma, anxiety, and the depression, the more its roots penetrate. But we can discover the healing modalities that help us to finally break covenant with these tormenters, flip the script and name it, speak it out, and take back control.

Because our stories matter.

Our emotional worlds matter. And sharing our voice isn't weakness.

It's how we survive.

This is how we change society and also our current medical system while reminding ourselves that we deserve to be heard and helped and believed, and are still worthy.

### *Suffering doesn't have to be our forever story.*

This is why your healing journey, whether it's from Medical PTSD or the depression, anxiety, or pain braided into all of it, has to be uniquely crafted for *you.* Not the glossy version of you other people want to see. Not for the "strong" persona you force yourself to wear day in and day out. But for the actual you, existing right now in this season, that is knee-deep in the emotional labor, the griefwork, the survival.

### *Healing is never linear. It's very personal, and it's holy work.*

I have personally tried countless therapies to help myself heal from Medical PTSD and anxiety from not only being literally run over by a truck but all of the traumas that followed since the diagnosis. And yes, so much in my life has improved. Absolutely. But there are still really challenging days, triggers that still pop up out of nowhere like a smell, a particular symptom, the sound of a loud engine, a location, or a tone in voice. And those triggers yank me immediately back into survival mode. And they remind me I am still a work in progress. That there is still so much more healing ahead.

And what worked for me won't necessarily work for you because healing in the area of our mental health isn't a one-size-fits-all equation. Your journey will become a tapestry of the pieces you collect along the way: the therapies, the boundaries, the rest, tears, the bodywork, tiny glimmers of hope, and the small, unexpected moments of joy.

And here is the thing about healing that might feel unbearably lonely but we need to remember: No one can do the healing *for* us. Of course, our loved ones can act as incredible cheerleaders, sending hilarious memes that make us snort when we want to crawl under a mound of blankets and hide from the world, praying for us, or just sitting with us in silence and holding our hands on the really dark days. Their presence matters so much.

But the inner place that we have to access? The unlearning of so much fear that has wrapped itself around our hearts and our brains? The slow rebuilding of trust within our own body?

That is solely ours.

And that body? This one precious, imperfect, stubborn yet beautiful body you inhabit?

Even in its exhaustion, even in its misfires, even in its chaos, your body has been fighting for you every single day. Carrying you through flares, bloodwork, hospital nights, missed diagnoses, frightening symptoms, and moments where you thought you wouldn't make it. Even when it gets it wrong, it is not your enemy. It is a determined, little warrior doing everything it can to maintain balance, recalibrate, find homeostasis, heal, and keep you here.

So, let's choose it back. Let's love on her. Let's offer her our attention. Our compassion. Our willingness to try, anything and everything. Consistently. Intentionally.

With patience. With grace.

Because this fierce yet gentle returning to ourselves is where our healing begins.

## CHAPTER 9

# BEYOND THE PILL BOTTLES: INTRODUCING THE ROOT & BLOOM PROTOCOL

The following sections explore a condensed version of The Root & Bloom Protocol—a protocol I've created over the years comprising treatments and therapies that go beyond conventional pharmaceuticals. While I've personally used many of these, this is not medical advice—please consult with a functional or integrative medicine provider to safely tailor anything to your unique needs, especially if you're on medication or have a complex diagnosis. And as I always tell my chronic illness community: Start low, go slow, and track everything.

Let's spill some truth that no influencer is sharing on their glittery Insta carousels: There isn't one single diet, cleanse, supplement, therapy, tea, or mystical smoothie that works for everyone who is living with chronic illness. If, amidst all the messages pumped your way daily through the internet, you feel confused or overwhelmed as you piece together the best healing route for you, you are in good company. It doesn't mean "everyone" else is getting it and you fell behind the curve. And it definitely doesn't mean you are missing out on the secret everyone else seems to know.

There is no secret.

There is no curve.

Creating a holistic healing plan that stretches far beyond the pill bottle isn't a straight line for anyone. It's more like a winding maze, full of occasional potholes and speedbumps. It's the culmination of thousands of hours of researching, experimenting, observing, and surviving trials and errors. As you walk on this path, you will find moments of hope and others that feel heartbreaking, especially when a therapy, supplement, or modality doesn't work.

But here's the beautiful part: This path will also provide you with incredible rewards—regaining energy, increasing a sense of agency, improving physical strength, and the hope-giving feeling of your life returning to you inch by inch.

I wish I could begin this chapter with the following: Here is the healing protocol, you're welcome. But we aren't living in influencer fantasyland. Here in the real world, figuring out your holistic path is messy. The emotional and financial toll is real. The options, while seemingly limitless, can also feel overwhelming. And it can feel scary when you are doing it alone. So, I want to walk this path with you, hand you the flashlight, and say: "Let's figure this one out together." No false promises. No lectures, just a companion on the road less traveled—the one that veers off from traditional pharma and into the terrain of integrative, holistic, and complementary healing.

I named the three-tier healing method I created while on my own journey, The Root & Bloom Protocol. It's based on what I discovered personally: Healing starts from the ground up, from the inside out, layer by layer. I believe the body already contains the knowledge to heal itself, but chronic illness can often scatter that signal. This three-tiered protocol, with two flexible sub tiers added in when you feel led, is designed to help you rebuild trust with your body and create the right environment for repair and healing.

It begins with foundational tools in Tier 1, like allergy, celiac, and stool testing, microbiome repair, gentle dietary shifts, and personalized adjustments you can often do at home. Tier 2 introduces advanced modalities such as mold and environmental toxin testing, functional medicine and supplementation, deeper herbology, lymph massage and acupuncture, ayurveda and more. And Tier 3 deepens the work with additional support through infrared and cryotherapy, IV nutrition, low dose naltrexone, hyperbaric and ozone therapy, and deeper detox work. The two sub tiers, which include spiritual or energetic work and trauma/nervous system support, can be added in at *any* point if and when you're ready.

This isn't a sprint, a cleanse, or a promise to "fix" you. The Root & Bloom Protocol won't return you to who you were before your diagnosis, because that's not the point. It's here to help you figure out what supports the version of you who exists now. The one waking up tired, inflamed, dismissed by doctors, and ready to try something different. You'll stack what works, discard what doesn't, pace what's overwhelming, and slowly collect tools that calm your body, reduce symptoms, and expand your capacity for joy.

But before we begin our journey into the protocol, I want to back up to where I first started and what set me on this path: Big Pharma.

Here's some truth: Even twenty-plus years into my diagnosis, some pharmaceuticals are still part of my daily routine. Every day. And, during certain life-threatening moments, pharmaceuticals have literally saved me. I honor that. I am grateful for that. But my hope that medications alone would carry me through or even cure my autoimmune diseases? That hope died a dramatic, fiery death somewhere around the mid-2000s.

That year, I was living in Fort Lauderdale, facing one of the worst lupus seasons of my life. After a particularly nasty flare, I wound up hospitalized for a time. The doctors' abilities seemed to have reached their limits. In that year, there was still not one drug specifically created and approved for lupus; instead, treatment consisted of drugs created for other diseases, particularly old chemotherapies, malaria drugs, and other medications that essentially shut off the immune system—like good ol' steroids, often called the Devil's tic-tacs in the chronic illness community. But nothing seemed to be working well. They sent me home from the hospital with the kind of shrug that says, *We've done everything we can. Now you wait.*

*But wait for what, exactly?* I thought. A miracle? Death? I didn't know. And honestly, I didn't have much energy to care.

I was slumped in a wheelchair day in and day out at home, the four corners of my living room becoming the borders of my entire universe. Getting upstairs or downstairs alone wasn't a reality. If my husband wasn't home and I was upstairs, I couldn't get myself food or water. So, we moved most of my belongings into that downstairs living room—my personal island of survival—for many, many months.

I was on over a dozen pharmaceutical medications at this time: some for lupus, others to manage the side effects of the initial medications, and somehow, I was getting worse.

Not plateauing. Not improving. *Worse.*

Eighty-seven pounds.

A sickly yellow coloring that would have been cute only if I were a banana.

And the unmistakable whisper in the back of my mind: *I'm dying. I can feel it.*

The little girl who once dreamed of changing the world and helping others? She was nowhere to be found. My world had shrunk to a recliner, a wheelchair, and the sound of my own breathing. I couldn't even dress myself. And then came the thought that changed everything:

If this doesn't course correct, Marisa, this will be the end of you.

The "end of me" felt unacceptable. Unthinkable. Even in my near-hopeless state, something in me snapped awake. A spark. A tiny ember beginning its burn. A whisper that said: "Absolutely not. Not yet, Marisa. Fight for your life or die trying."

Passively accepting that my body was giving up was not an option for me. I was pumped up mentally and ready to break agreements with any life-depleting beliefs I had succumbed to—the "I'm never going to get better" to all forms of "My life is over." I refused to disappear inside of my illness and die but where in the actual world does someone begin when they can barely sit upright? When breathing takes up the bulk of someone's energy each day?

It was pre-smartphone explosion, pre-wellness influencer revolution, pre-basically-everything-at-your-fingertips land. There were no such things as apps or online practitioners or health coaches sliding into my DMs with discount codes. What I *did* have, though, was a computer, books, and a limited section of new video streaming capabilities thanks to Netflix and YouTube. And for reasons I still can't fully explain, that's where it all started for me.

And with the thought, *There has to be more than these medications, right?,* in the back of my mind, I began consuming documentaries and books like they were air. Soon after, came experiments in my own kitchen and in time and when my wallet allowed, working one-on-one with practitioners that worked outside of the traditional Western Medicine box.

In a nutshell, that was the beginning of my holistic health journey. And it's the imperfect, emotional, but ultimately empowering path I want to help you begin too.

## Brick By Brick

Before we dive into a condensed version of my Root & Bloom Protocol, there is an exercise I want you to consider: Pick a mantra. Find one below that resonates or use one as a springboard and create your own. I know, I know, *This is so cheesy, Marisa!* And it may seem that way, but there is a legitimate reason behind this exercise. As you walk this journey, which could be months, years, or honestly, life-long, there will be days you absolutely want to quit. Days when you don't see any progress in the natural realm. Days when the supplements feel scammy and super expensive. And days when your body legitimately feels like a full-time research experiment and the alternative therapy seems totally pointless.

And this is why a mantra is crucial. It will be the anchor you return to again and again. A reminder that you are so worth this journey, the effort, the financial investment, the time, and the healing. We are going to think of this mantra as our seatbelt that buckles us in and keeps us grounded when the terrain is rocky AF.

I love you enough to tell you the truth: Bringing healing to certain areas of your life will be one of the hardest things you've ever done. And remember, nothing we are about to discuss is meant to be taken as, "take this" or "try that" and *you'll be completely healed.* The healing I'm talking about is found over time. It's adding tools to your toolbox that start to lessen symptoms—maybe giving you a few stronger days each week instead of none. It's waking up at a level 4 pain instead of a 10 and letting that shift compound. One thing stacks on another, and little by little, you start to gain more bandwidth—and with it, you begin gaining pieces of your life back.

Here are a few mantras to consider:

"I refuse to abandon myself. Even on the really hard days, especially on those days, I am worth fighting for."

"Progress isn't always visible or speedy. But I am showing up, and showing up is healing too."

"My body is not the enemy here. It is trying to fight everyday, and I will keep choosing it and fighting alongside it, breath after breath."

And my personal favorite:

"I will not give up on my body. I will not give up on my future; this is not where my story ends."

Found one that resonates? Perfect. Write it on a Post-it and then slap it to your bathroom mirror. Make it your phone's wallpaper. Tattoo it on your heart (metaphorically speaking). And voice it openly on a regular basis. Truth: Our cells respond to the things we say.

Now, let's get to work.

I'm going to take a wild guess here, but I'm assuming most of you do *not* have a money tree flourishing in your backyard. (If you do, please send me a seed immediately!). And for many of us, the road to diagnosis alone has already drained much of our bank accounts, our energy reserves, and perhaps a bit of our sanity. Staying afloat while being sick, especially if you are unable to work or living solely off an assistance program, adds another layer of financial strain that no one warned us about.

And while building a holistic healing path will take some investment, hear me clearly: You do not have to try everything at once, empty your savings, or turn your kitchen into a full-time research lab unless you want to—I sort of did at one point. In fact, I urge you not to try "all the things" listed below at once. It won't work; your body isn't physically ready for it, you'll have a hell of a time differentiating what is working vs. what isn't, plus, it will emotionally overwhelm you. Healing is not a race to accumulate the most therapies; it's a slow layering of what actually supports *your* body.

If any of the options we discuss below intrigue you, start with one small thing.

Just one.

Try it. Sit with it. Watch it.

And while you're doing that one new thing, take notes each time. Copious notes. Or voice memos and video diaries if writing isn't your jam. (Yes, this is me revisiting my earlier sermon about journaling; we've come full circle.) Track whether something helps, does nothing, or makes things worse. Track the small wins and the subtle shifts, in addition to the times you don't feel any change whatsoever.

This isn't busywork. This is data. *Your* data.

And this becomes the architectural blueprint, the healing path, of the new home your body is becoming.

Why Three Tiers?

We're about to dive into a lot of information like, "make a pot of tea and clear your afternoon" levels of information. To keep it manageable and to avoid your nervous system quietly leaving the chat, I've broken this protocol into three main tiers, plus two optional sub-tiers you can plug in whenever you're ready. Maybe you're still in Tier 1 but curious about a modality from a sub-tier—go for it. Or maybe you wait until Tier 3 before adding in sub-tier options. It all depends on your physical and emotional readiness, your energy levels, your wallet, and frankly, what lights you up. This is the roadmap I personally followed, but I fully encourage you to cherry-pick your own path based on what fits *your* life, not mine.

And not to nag, but a gentle reiteration, please take your time with this or any protocol you choose; this was a multi-year process for me and I still add in new treatments, therapies/supplements as the years go by. Healing isn't linear and it definitely isn't a race. Each approach takes time to show signs of improvement (or no improvement), and that's okay. Remember, this is about creating deep roots that will carry you long-term, not checking boxes.

# CHAPTER 10

# THE ROOT & BLOOM PROTOCOL TIER 1: ROOT

Lay the groundwork, uncover data, begin nutritional and gut healing options.

As we move into the three tiers, I consider Tier 1 the root—the base layer of healing from which everything else grows. While some of the tools across the protocol may feel time-consuming or tough depending on your current physical state, Tier 1 offers some of the most accessible, doable entry points that can still spark real shifts. And the best part? Most of it can be done right from home—which, let's be honest, is probably where you're spending most of your time if you're navigating chronic illness. This tier is about grounding, gathering data, and gently setting the conditions your body needs to begin rebuilding. No pressure, no rush—just root down and start where you are.

It may seem odd, but I often start Root conversations in the area of allergies. I believe there is a deep understanding necessary to the role allergies and sensitivities play, in addition to a crucial need to know what your body specifically dislikes. As I briefly mentioned earlier, there is immense research available indicating that patients with inflammatory diseases and autoimmune issues often have coexisting allergic conditions, with the newest research showing these chronic conditions and allergies actually share overlapping pathogenic pathways.[1] Of course, even those with other chronic conditions that aren't autoimmune in nature (and also our "healthies" out there), can all suffer some type of allergic issue. In fact, the Center for Disease Control estimates over 100 million Americans over the age of eighteen deal with some form of allergic issue, whether seasonal allergies, food allergies, or eczema, making allergy on its own a chronic illness.[2]

The reason I begin here is because having unidentified allergies can trigger inflammation and make a variety of symptoms worse. If you do not know what you are sensitive or allergic to, how can you ever come up with a safe dietary plan or know what supplements or therapies are a lower risk option for your body? *You can't.* Without this knowledge, adding that "healthy" food that everyone swears by to your plate or ingesting a supplement with a filler ingredient that can trigger symptoms can do more harm than good.

I emphasize this because allergic reactions—when you don't know what's triggering them—can completely derail your healing path and make you feel like you're losing both your mind *and* your progress. I've been dealing with food and environmental allergies since I was basically in diapers. Throw in lifelong asthma and an instantaneous emotional attachment to every furry animal I'm allergic to, and yeah—it's been a real party. Understanding your allergic landscape early on can save you a lot of confusion, flares, and unintentional backtracking.

Here's something to be aware of: If you've had the same allergy panel since high school taped to your fridge and are using it as your

Master Guide to safe foods, note that allergies can shift over time.[3] I wish someone had told me that earlier; it would've saved me a lot of frustration and "why is my body doing this?" moments.

So, there I was, deep in the clean-eating trenches, working with nutritionists, reading every label like it held government secrets, and still feeling awful. I'd started with food on my "healing path" because it felt doable: I had control over it, it was already in my house, and hey, I loved to cook and had to eat every day anyway, so why not start there? But, spoiler alert: Food control doesn't equal food clarity. Especially when you're guessing and not working with real-time evidence. And soon enough, two specific issues made me recognize why it would be crucial to have said evidence.

During that season, two unexpected issues crashed the party and sent me straight to an out-of-the-box allergist in my area—a total superhero of a woman who, thankfully, was always willing to explore both traditional medicine and alternative options. We slowly worked our way through a mountain of testing but it all started with two major red flags.

First, I developed chronic spontaneous urticaria, and by that I mean hundreds of angry welts erupted across my body out of nowhere, swelling my eyes shut and leaving a trail of hives from my face to my feet. It was one of the scariest moments of my life. I genuinely thought, *if lupus didn't take me out, this might.* The second issue? Out of the blue, I started experiencing relentless stomach problems; this was bizarre because I had what my family lovingly called a "steel stomach." I was the person who could throw back a bowl of pepperoncini and roasted garlic everyday like it was a light snack. So, when even bland, benign foods started triggering symptoms, I knew something had shifted.

That kicked off what was, at the time, considered the gold standard of allergy testing: pressure testing, patch tests, full back/skin tests, blood panels, and even the dreaded oral consumption challenges (a.k.a., eat-this-and-pray-nothing-happens test). My allergist and I were determined to figure it out, and we took the long, winding route to get there, but it gave us real answers I couldn't have gotten anywhere else.

Most of my allergens were the usual suspects I'd carried since childhood: sky-high reactions to dust, animals, seafood . . . you know, the greatest hits. But then came the surprise twist. The skin tests confirmed what we were starting to see in the bloodwork: Some of the foods I loved most—including the avocados I was eating once or twice a day like it was my full-time job—were now showing up as problematic. Same with several of the fresh fruits and vegetables I practically lived on (because honestly, they're my favorite food group).

But here's where it gets nuanced: these were sensitivities. Meaning, they weren't sending me into anaphylaxis like shellfish would (that one's still a hard no unless I'm trying to meet my maker). Instead, these "healthy" foods were quietly wreaking havoc on my digestion and adding to my inflammation every single day without me realizing it.

It's crucial to understand the difference here before you run off and make your food plan. Food *allergies* trigger an immediate immune system response—often severe or even life-threatening, think trouble breathing, swelling, drop in blood pressure. Sensitivities and intolerances, on the other hand, often cause delayed, low-grade reactions, think bloating, fatigue, brain fog, a skin blotch here or there, or GI issues—uncomfortable, yes, but not necessarily fatal. Learning what I was allergic to, and sensitive to, changed how I looked at everything I was putting on my plate.

So there I was, eating *so* healthy. Combatting inflammation: woohoo! Getting those good fats in? Check! And literally making myself sicker in the process because I was introducing items every day to a body that couldn't tolerate them, causing a histamine overload just coursing through my body. And I had no clue why I wasn't feeling better—blotchy, itchy, 24/7 stomachaches, and more fatigue than normal. I just kept beating myself up mentally thinking, *everything on my plate is so healthy, why isn't it working? Maybe I need to eat more of it?* Strike!

Once I finally knew exactly what needed to be cut out at least for a season, I was in the best possible position to actually begin. With that clarity, my nutritionist and I built a safe, personalized meal plan, and more importantly, started identifying which ingredients in supplements and even some medications I needed to avoid like the plague.

This is exactly why I'm stressing this as your true starting line—because without these foundational insights, you're just planting seeds in dry soil. You're guessing, flaring, and spinning your wheels instead of rooting your healing in something solid. And let's be real: No one with chronic illness has time or energy for that kind of chaos.

## Tier I: Root

### *Identifying Allergies, Sensitivities, and Intolerances*

1. Start by finding an allergist in your area who can test you for both food and environmental allergies and sensitivities using the methods we've already discussed: skin prick tests, patch testing, blood work, and if needed oral food challenges. These tests can give you crucial insight into what your immune system is reacting to.

2. If you live in a rural area, don't have insurance, or are working with a tight budget, there are at-home food sensitivity kits available from reputable companies. These usually involve a small blood or hair sample, and while they aren't as comprehensive as what an allergist can provide, they're a helpful starting point. Just remember: Most of these online kits only test for sensitivities, *not* true IgE-mediated allergies, so they're not a replacement for clinical allergy testing if you suspect severe reactions.
3. While you're getting tested for allergens, ask your allergist or primary care provider about screening for celiac disease, an autoimmune disorder triggered by gluten.
4. Diagnosing celiac can start with bloodwork—here are the key markers:

- tTG-IgA (Tissue Transglutaminase IgA)
- Total IgA
- EMA-IgA (Endomysial Antibody IgA)
- Deamidated Gliadin Peptide (DGP) IgA/IgG

These tests can often be run through standard labs, but at-home kits for celiac screening are also available if getting to a clinic isn't doable. Personally, I believe blood testing is a valuable first step, especially if you're not physically or financially ready to jump straight into a GI referral and endoscopy under sedation to collect intestinal biopsies, which Western medicine deems the gold standard for diagnosis. This approach lets you rule in or rule out key triggers early on without immediately going invasive.

### *Implementing Your Findings into Your Dietary Protocols*

Once you've got actual evidence in hand about what your body loves, hates, and barely tolerates when it comes to food and allergens, you can finally stop guessing and start building a plan that works for *your* body. No more spinning the wheel of random elimination diets or blaming the kale. In the chronic illness community, we hear a lot of diet names thrown around—some helpful, some hype-y. I've tried almost all of them, some with great success.

Let's take a look at the most common ones you'll come across and may want to consider:

- **Autoimmune Protocol (AIP)/Elimination:** A strict elimination diet designed to calm autoimmune inflammation by removing the most common allergic triggers such as: dairy, grains, eggs, nightshades, etc. then slowly reintroducing foods to identify sensitivities. It focuses on nutrient-dense, gut-healing foods to support immune balance.
- **Carnivore:** This all-animal product diet (meat, organs, fat) eliminates plant foods and grains to reduce inflammation, gut irritation, and immune triggers in people with severe sensitivities or autoimmune flares.
- **Vegetarian**: A plant-based diet that excludes meat and fish, it is potentially rich in antioxidants and fiber to support gut health and lower inflammation, but requires thoughtful planning to meet protein and nutrient needs in chronic illness.
- **LowFODMAP:** This is created as a short-term diet that reduces fermentable sugars (FODMAPs) found in certain fruits, vegetables, grains, and dairy to alleviate bloating, pain,

and digestive symptoms common in IBS and chronic gut disorders.

- **Low Histamine:** This protocol is designed to avoid high-histamine foods like aged cheeses, fermented items, and leftovers that can trigger flares in people with histamine intolerance or Mast Cell Activation Syndrome (MCAS), reducing allergy-like or inflammatory symptoms.
- **Anti-Inflammatory:** A flexible eating pattern focused on whole, unprocessed foods—rich in fruits, vegetables, omega-3s, and healthy fats—that supports immune regulation and reduces chronic inflammation across a wide range of illnesses.
- **Anti-Candida Diet:** A low-sugar, low-yeast eating plan aimed at starving Candida yeast overgrowth in the gut. This overgrowth is believed to contribute to fatigue, brain fog, bloating, and immune issues. It removes sugar, refined carbs, alcohol, and often fermented foods, while emphasizing non-starchy vegetables, lean proteins, and antifungal support.
- **Juicing:** Juicing involves extracting juice from vegetables, fruits, and herbs to deliver a concentrated dose of vitamins, minerals, and antioxidants with minimal digestive effort. For those with chronic illness, it can support hydration, reduce inflammation, and gently assist detoxification, especially helpful when appetite or digestion is impaired. Juices should be made with minimal fruit to avoid blood sugar spikes, as well as tailored to individual fruit/vegetable sensitivities.

Which one is right for you? Only you can decide. This is where I would suggest working with an experienced professional familiar with your specific diagnosis, allergies, and goals. It may not be one of these diets in particular. It may be combining different elements of various diets to create your own unique food protocol. While I have had incredible success in lowering pharmaceutical medication amounts and decreasing symptoms using elements of juicing, carnivore, and anti-inflammatory diet aspects, and healed from leaky-gut symptoms using elimination diet protocols for short periods of time, you may see improvement by incorporating autoimmune protocol and anti-Candida elements, depending on your health challenges.

I fully understand that not everyone has the ability to work with a nutritionist, functional medicine doctor, or health coach and if that's you right now, you can still move forward. It just means you'll need to take on the role of researcher, detective, and test subject at one time. Start by diving into credible resources—I'm talking books, podcasts, and online communities focused on the dietary approach that seems most aligned with your symptoms and needs. Many of these protocols have free meal plans, grocery guides, and budget-friendly hacks shared by others who've walked the same path. Instagram, Pinterest, and Reddit may not be medical journals, but they're goldmines of lived experience when you're starting from scratch. You'll find scores of patient communities talking about testing kits, top tier books, practitioner recommendations, and more.

Once you pick a starting point—whether it's elements of AIP, anti-inflammatory, low histamine, or something else—commit to it for a few weeks to a few months, depending on the protocol. During that time, *track everything*: how you feel after meals, your digestion, mood, energy, skin, sleep, weight, even blood sugar (if you're able). Look for patterns, document flares, and be willing to tweak as you go.

My own dietary journey has evolved over two decades; sometimes I circle back to protocols that worked in the past when I hit a flare or when symptoms start creeping back in after I've gone off-course (hello, travel snacks and absent health food stores when you are traveling in the boondocks).

If you're starting with an elimination diet or LowFODMAP, know this: These types of diets are meant to be short-term tools, not your forever. Yes, it may feel like you're giving up your beloved foods but think of it as a temporary investigation. It's a targeted experiment designed to give you actual answers—what's triggering you, what's calming you, and how to move toward a more sustainable, customized way of eating that supports healing instead of guessing. You've got this, and you don't need a white coat to start figuring it out.

### *Next Steps: Concentrating on the Microbiome*

Just like a plant can't thrive in depleted soil, your body can't thrive without a balanced, nourished gut. And so, you must take a closer look at the microbiome before diving fully into your dietary protocol of choice, because you will not be able to fully benefit from the nutrition protocol if your gut microbiome is not in a state where it can absorb and process nutrients and utilize what you're eating.

The microbiome is the inner ecosystem of the gut and contains literally trillions of bacteria, fungi, and other microbes. These microbes digest food, produce critical vitamins, regulate your immune system, and even communicate with your brain. When the microbiome is in disarray, an all-too-common reality when someone is chronically ill, even the "healthiest" and most ideal dietary protocol won't be as successful as you hoped.

What are the signs *your* microbiome may be off kilter? If you are bloated after you eat, suddenly reacting to random foods, dealing with high pain levels, experiencing reflux and indigestion, having issues with your bowel movements, and dealing with fatigue that just won't quit, your gut is waving *all* the red flags, my friend. And the truth? Unless the microbiome is fully addressed, *no* individualized dietary protocol will work to its potential. End of story.

What kinds of tools can detect if your microbiome is out of whack? First stop: a comprehensive stool test. And no, I'm *not* talking about the standard one you get from your family doctor. When I say *this sh**t is different, I mean it literally and figuratively. Most conventional stool tests in the US barely scratch the surface, checking for a small handful of pathogens at best. And that is even if you can find a MD in the USA that will request one for you. What you need is an at-home testing kit that analyzes your entire gut terrain like a microbial crime scene.

These tests go deep (no pun intended), looking at your levels of good and bad bacteria, both aerobic and anaerobic, yeast, fungi, inflammation markers, Candida, signs of H. pylori, fat and protein digestion, and even evidence that you may have been exposed to mold (more on that delightful topic later). Many of these tests also examine things like leaky gut markers (called Zonulin markers), parasitic activity, and overall diversity of your microbiome. It's basically a health report card for your gut, and guess what: most of us are flunking.

While I'm not affiliated with any of the following companies, I've personally used several and found their reports and recommendations eye-opening and genuinely helpful in creating a plan that made sense. A few solid options are Verisana, Viome, and Tiny Health, all of which can be ordered without begging a doctor for a lab slip. If you prefer to get it done in a physical lab, Walkinlab.com also offers an array of stool tests you can book and complete at a local lab, no white coat signature required.

Depending on your results, your next move will likely include feeding and rebalancing your microbes. Here are a few to consider researching or mentioning to your nutritionist and functional medicine practitioner:

- **Prebiotics** such as garlic, leeks, asparagus, dandelion root, etc. are the fibrous plant materials that feed good bacteria. Prebiotics can also be supplemented via powders, capsules, and gummies.
- **Probiotics** are the live bacteria themselves, either from fermented foods if tolerated or supplements.
- **Postbiotics** are the beneficial compounds those bacteria produce once they're thriving—like short-chain fatty acids that reduce inflammation.

* *A note about any of the above: You may need to start extremely slow with these as you begin your holistic journey (especially probiotics, which can cause flares in some sensitive systems), but building a foundation here is crucial if you want lasting change.*

### Additional Gut Repair Remedy: Homemade Bone Broth

One of my absolutely tried and true at home remedies that is both nourishing and low-effort in supporting your gut lining and microbiome is homemade bone broth. I'm talking about simmering a variety of bones in your crockpot or via stovetop for twelve to twenty-four hours with water, apple cider vinegar, vegetables (carrots and celery are most common) and spices. Whichever herbs you decide to add can be dependent upon your specific needs and/or symptoms, but some of the most often used include rosemary, ginger, thyme, garlic, nettle, astragalus root, and turmeric with black pepper. Here is a quick break down-on what each spice and herb can add to your bone broth as far as healing properties:

- **Rosemary:** Rich in antioxidants and anti-inflammatory compounds
- **Ginger:** Adds a kick of warm spicy flavor, and helps with inflammation and overall digestion
- **Oregano:** Has antifungal properties
- **Thyme:** Can boost immune support through antioxidants and anti-inflammatory polyphenols like thymol
- **Garlic:** Adds robust flavor, plus anti-inflammatory and immune boosting properties
- **Nettle Leaf/Root:** A superfood packed with vitamins and minerals
- **Astragalus Root:** A medicinal herb that supports immune function
- **Turmeric:** Adds color, and has anti-inflammatory properties that are increased when paired with black pepper

### Bone Broth

Simmering bones for a long period of time extracts collagen, gelatin, and amino acids, which all help rebuild and are soothing to the gut lining. Sipping a warm cup on a chilly day is to me truly an act of self-care. I also use the broth as my base for soups and whenever I cook rice, quinoa, or oat porridge.

While bone broth might feel like trendy wellness Instagram advice, I promise you its benefits are vast. For many years, it has continued to calm my digestion, help me heal from leaky gut symptoms, and become my go-to nutrient-source during severe flares when eating a meal is absolutely not possible. While it is not a cure-all, I like to think of it as one of my many grounding practices that helps me feel like I am working alongside my body in our healing.

### *Adding in a Gut Powerhouse:*

**L-glutamine**

If you feel specific gut issues are an ongoing issue or you are just dedicated to improving your overall gut health, I would mention L-glutamine to your nutritionist and/or functional medicine doctor if you're working with one. L–glutamine is a powerhouse when it comes to healing the gut lining, assisting in repairing the microbiome, and helping your immune system fight germs.

Here's why L-glutamine should be considered: Gut Lining Repair. What's the most abundant of the twenty different L-glutamine—take a bow, you understated little superhero.[4] When your gut lining gets damaged from stress, flares, infections, meds, you name it, things that are not supposed to leave your intestines like toxins, undigested food, and microbes, start slipping into your bloodstream. This is what people mean when they talk about "leaky gut," and it's a major trigger for inflammation, autoimmune activity, and allergic reactions. If the AIP diet discussed above interests you, you'll see it's intertwined with helping to heal leaky gut as you eliminate certain inflammatory foods and allow repair of the gut lining. When you use L-glutamine, think of it as stepping in to help seal the cracks by fueling those delicate gut wall cells and supporting tighter junctions, making it a foundational tool in rebuilding your barrier function from the inside out.

L-glutamine comes in a couple of easy-to-use forms—powder or capsules—and I'm personally a big fan of Metagenics' L-glutamine powder and honestly, their whole supplement line which I obtain through my functional medicine doctor. This particular amino acid has made a huge difference in both my gut health and my allergy symptoms. Over time, I was even able to reintroduce some of the fruits and vegetables I'd previously been sensitive to—a big win in my book as my diet is fairly limited as it is.

That said, always do your own research before adding new supplements to your routine, and if possible, work with a practitioner who understands both your diagnosis *and* your goals. High doses of L-glutamine aren't right for everyone—especially those with liver or kidney disease, Reye's Syndrome, or seizure disorders like epilepsy.

**Medicinal Mushrooms**

Let's talk fungi—potentially your gut's new best friend! Medicinal mushrooms are becoming increasingly popular, popping up in coffees, protein powders, teas, and tinctures. Some hard hitters include reishi, lion's mane, and turkey tail. Various medicinal mushrooms have been used for centuries in traditional Eastern medicine to support immune function and feed beneficial gut bacteria.[5] Modern science and research now back this up, as it's been discovered that medical mushrooms literally feed beneficial gut bacteria, promoting growth and helping to balance the gut microbiota.[6]

While mushrooms provide a variety of immune benefits, not everyone should "dig" in. If you have mold allergies, histamine intolerance, or certain fungal sensitivities, mushrooms may trigger symptoms or overwhelm your system. They also need to be used with caution in people with diabetes, certain autoimmune and liver conditions, as well as those pregnant or breastfeeding. When in doubt about adding mushrooms to your regimen, work with a practitioner who has deep insight on *both mushrooms and mast cells* and begin very slowly with a method where it's easier to control the dosage (think highly diluted tinctures).

**Butyrate**

Ah, butyrate—the perfect name for something related to your colon, no? While it's not exactly sexy, this short-chain fatty acid is another big shot when it comes to improving your gut health. The easiest way to describe it? Gut fuel. Butyrate is produced in your colon when your gut bacteria ferment certain types of fiber. It plays a major role in keeping your intestinal lining strong, your inflammation low, and digestion running smoothly.[7]

It helps heal leaky gut, supports immune function, and may even reduce colon cancer risk, and improve brain-gut signaling (yes, the microbes are running the whole show). If ongoing, erratic GI symptoms have been plaguing you, you might want to consider low butyrate production playing a role especially if you've taken a lot of antibiotics, have a limited diet, or your gut microbiome has taken some serious hits due to stress, infections, etc. In fact, research shows lower levels of butyrate are continuously found to be linked to specific GI conditions including Inflammatory Bowel Disease, colorectal cancer, and gut inflammation.[8]

Now for the good part: Did you know you can boost butyrate naturally in your very own kitchen through food? This is a great option if the thought of taking another supplement causes an involuntary eye roll. Your gut microbes make butyrate when you eat resistant starches:

think cold cooked potatoes (basically, the food is fully cooked then refrigerated), oats that have been soaked overnight (hello, Pinterest overnight oats recipes!), green bananas, and legumes. Regular rotation of these foods in your menu offers you an ideal and natural way to boost this fatty acid.

You might be wondering, why do I need to cool the food after it's cooked? Well, the food's resistant starch content increases when cooled, which your bacteria love to devour and then they pay you back in butyrate as a thank-you gift.

**Digestive Bitters: The Often-Forgotten Digestive Superpower**

Long before there were shelves of digestive enzyme capsules or antacids, there were plants, and bitter plants at that. From these plants, cultures across the world have spent thousands of years crafting what we now call digestive bitters. You'll still find them in practice today—from Traditional Chinese Medicine to European herbalism to Ayurveda—all rooted in one core principle: Bitter flavors wake up your digestive system and get things moving.

When you taste something bitter, and I mean *truly* bitter, not "ooh this mushroom tastes earthy," it actually triggers a reflex through your vagus nerve that tells your brain: "Hey Chief! Fire up the GI engines." This stimulates stomach acid production, bile flow from the liver and gallbladder, and digestive enzymes. Simply put: Bitters help your body prepare to break down and absorb your food *before* you even take the first bite, which is crucial when you're dealing with bloating, sluggish digestion, SIBO (Small Intestinal Bacterial Overgrowth), or microbial imbalance issues.

So, what exactly is *in* digestive bitters? Some of the most common herbs include:

- **Dandelion root:** Which can gently detox your liver while also supporting flow of bile.
- **Artichoke leaf:** Aids in digesting fat and also supports the liver.
- **Gentian root:** Stimulates digestive activity and is known for its extreme bitterness.
- **Citrus and orange peel:** Can aid in digestion and help relieve bloating and gas.
- **Chamomile:** Can calm spasms and soothe the GI tract.
- **Fennel:** Relaxes GI muscles, improves flow of digestive fluids, and can lessen gas and cramping.
- **Angelica root:** Stimulates stomach acid and the secretion of bile and can help in the breakdown of heavy meals.

Though I didn't know it at the time, I used digestive bitters successfully as a child, as my grandparents would give them to me whenever I complained of a stomachache (almost daily as the typical Italian diet—wheat and cheese—was trying to take me out three times a day). Today, you can find reputable brands that offer tinctures made from organic and wildcrafted herbs. In time, if herbs interest you as much as they do me, you may want to consider classes or training with an herbal field guide to discover how to harvest and identify safe plant parts to make your own tinctures.

In my opinion, bitters are one of the simplest, oldest, and most overlooked digestive tools out there. For some of us living chronically ill, they can be the key to getting the upper digestive system back online and moving along—which then helps prevent microbial chaos further down the GI tract. It's not about popping more pills *after* your meal; it's about retraining your body how to digest food again, from the top down.

If you feel you are extremely sensitive to medication, herbs, and supplements, start at the lowest serving possible, and under the supervision of a professional. Keep in mind, bitters are not for everyone with a chronic illness. Avoid them if you have active ulcers and gastritis, blocked bile ducts or gallstones, severe gastric reflux, have mast cell or histamine issues, or are pregnant/nursing.

**Targeted Herbal Antimicrobials (For Dysbiosis or Overgrowth)**

While we're on one of my favorite topics—herbal allies—let's pivot to an important condition to be aware of: SIBO or Small Intestinal Bacterial Overgrowth: a gut condition that may be flying under the radar if your symptoms are more severe or resistant to change. SIBO happens when bacteria that are supposed to live happily in your large intestine decide they want to move to a new living space, a.k.a. your small intestine, where they absolutely do *not* belong.

When this occurs, you feel the shift in the form of bloating, gas, pain, constipation, diarrhea, food reactions, fatigue, and even brain fog. We hear about SIBO more in recent years, and research shows it tends to overlap with people who have been diagnosed with autoimmune disease, fibromyalgia, or IBS, or have a long history of antibiotic use or abdominal surgeries.[9]

One common way SIBO is diagnosed is through a breath test, which you *can* request from your family doctor or GI specialist, but if they stare at you blankly or claim SIBO isn't "a real issue to be concerned with," you can also order at-home kits from places like TrioSmartBreath or the Institute for Digestive Wellbeing.

Depending on your test result, here is where herbs re-enter the scene: One of the most common ways to combat SIBO, other than antibiotics, is through anti-microbial herbal extracts. Depending on the anti-microbial regimen you decide on, you can expect concoctions to contain herbs like oregano oil, berberine, neem, garlic extract, black walnut, feverfew, skullcap, and allicin—as a gentler alternative to prescription antibiotics. You can even look into alternative herbal antibiotic therapies from the following companies:

- Candibactin-AR® and Candibactin-BR® from Metagenics
- FC-Cidal™ and Dysbiocide® from Biotics Research
- Biocidin from Biocidin Botanicals

The overall goal of these herbs is to reduce the overgrowth without wiping out your entire microbiome. Protocols may vary in length but typically range around several weeks. In addition, many protocols alternate combinations every two weeks to avoid bacterial resistance, and pair them with a motility aid like fresh ginger or Iberogast and a low-fermentation diet such as LowFODMAP, as this temporarily reduces the amount of fermentable carbohydrates that these misplaced gut bacteria love to feed and grow on.

My biggest caveats with SIBO? First, it can be tricky to treat, and I want you to know that going in, so you don't panic if it doesn't vanish in a week or so. Second, go slow and *track every single response* to whatever protocol you choose. Some people experience what's called a "die-off reaction"—basically, as the bacteria die (peace out, guys!), they release toxins that can temporarily make you feel pretty terrible (think bloating, fatigue, brain fog, or flu-like symptoms). But these die-off symptoms aren't a sign things aren't working but rather a sign your body is reacting to the protocol.

The key is pacing, not quitting. Untreated SIBO can lead to nutrient malabsorption, higher inflammation, and worsening immune dysfunction—all the stuff we're trying to calm down. Bottom line: SIBO is a tough little gremlin— stubborn and absolutely capable of boomeranging back. If possible, work with a practitioner to tailor treatment to your body's speed and needs, so you can knock it out for good!

Last and certainly not least, though I haven't personally tried it yet, there has been a lot of chatter in my inner spoonie circle lately about frequency-activated nano silver for optimizing gut health, destroying harmful invaders and also helping to support the immune system. It is believed frequency-activated silver dismantles the protection system (cell walls) or gut invaders, essentially dismantling them without interrupting your beneficial gut bacteria.

## Tier 1 Wrap-Up: Look at You Laying Down Roots!

Each tier of this protocol is an experiment: one that might take months, or even a year, before you're ready to layer in more from the next tier. When that time comes, hit pause and do a quick "garden" inventory:

- What therapies or tools from Tier 1 actually helped your energy, symptoms, mental clarity, or overall feeling of wellbeing?
- Which ones flopped, felt off, or made things worse—and why?
- Most importantly, which ones earned a spot in your master "gardener toolbox" as you move forward?

This isn't busywork—it's building your own personalized healing manual. I did the same thing during my journey, and years later, I still lean on my master list every day or switch back to specific protocols I know work during a flare. With every tier, you'll keep adding tools, refining, and ultimately creating a protocol that's made *just* for your body, allowing you to ultimately bloom.

## CHAPTER 11

# THE ROOT & BLOOM PROTOCOL TIER 2: GROW

Your roots are down and you have made it to Tier 2. You've weeded through allergens, planted some dietary structure, maybe even befriended a probiotic or two. Now comes Tier 2: Grow—and it's time to expand the garden. In this phase, you'll start to explore things that dig a little deeper into the healing realm: functional medicine, strategic supplementation through medical-grade products, considering hidden environmental stressors like mold and metals, cleansing your home and body of petrochemicals, and supporting drainage pathways.

It's a little more advanced than Tier 1, but it's also where some people really start to see increased movement, feel even less symptomatic, and more connected to their body. Just like in real gardening, growth takes tending—not speed. So, pace yourself with the modalities and therapies in Tier 2 just as you did in Tier 1. And don't forget to keep copious notes so you can look back at this tier and know exactly what worked for you and in what ways you enjoyed the fruits (less symptoms, more energy, etc.) of your labor.

Tier 2 is where we start getting into the nitty-gritty—and that often means teaming up with a functional medicine practitioner or coach. If you found one back in Tier 1, great! If not, this is a good time to explore your options locally or virtually. And here's a pro-tip: In the US, many chiropractors moonlight as functional medicine pros thanks to extra education and training. If the term functional medicine is new to you, it is essentially a doctor who focuses on identifying and correcting the root causes of illness (often through personalized lifestyle, nutrition, and lab analysis) rather than primarily prescribing medication to manage symptoms. Functional medicine is finally getting its long overdue moment—and chiropractors are often a more affordable route but in all honesty, appointments and supplements still do add up.

When I first started working with a functional medicine doctor, I didn't have an unlimited health budget. So he and I struck a rhythm: long, meaty appointments every few months where we'd cover a half dozen steps: supplement ideas, gentle interventions, possible next directions, and then I'd go off on my own to test and track what worked. He was a gem and answered every anxious question, concern or possible side effect I had along the way, but I know not everyone has that kind of access. Luckily, there are now many functional medicine providers and coaches who work virtually and can help you build a plan from wherever you are, no road trip required.

One of the biggest shifts you'll see in the protocols listed in this tier is a focus on stronger supplementation and deeper herbology. I am talking about *medical-grade supplements*: High-quality vitamins and nutrients produced under strict standards for purity and potency (think: pharma-level quality, minus well, everything that comes with pharma), that are third-party tested and use top-tier ingredients that are continuously checked for mold, metals, and other contaminants. These supplements are designed for better bioavailability—meaning your body might actually *use* them instead of just . . . escorting them out (truth: Many drugstore supplements use cheap ingredients that are not easily utilized by the body and may not be tested for contaminants).

Some of the trusted medical-grade supplement brands I started with years ago and still use today include Metagenics, Standard Process, Pure Encapsulations, Integrative Therapeutics, and Thorne. The good news is you can get your hands on many of these now without needing a practitioner's permission slip. Medical-grade supplementation without gatekeeping? Yes baby, accessibility has *finally* entered the chat!

Now, let's dig in.

## Tier 2: Grow

Go deeper with advanced modalities and therapies to help you thrive.

Before digging into functional medicine's medical-grade supplementation, there are specific tests your practitioner will likely want to run. These can help tailor specific supplementation and therapies to deficiencies, inflammatory markers, metabolic issues, etc. and will help you discover your baseline so you can compare your results before and after supplementation/therapies. Don't forget, if any of these tests interest you but you are not able to work directly with a practitioner, you can order many of these or similar tests yourself through online labs such as Any Lab Test Now, LabCorp on Demand, Direct Labs and Persona Labs among many others.

In addition, there are many biotech companies in recent years that offer extensive advanced and specialty biomarker health memberships that perform over 100 blood and/or saliva tests. These are typically annual membership types of plans, but in many cases are cheaper than completing this bloodwork individually through a lab (for those without insurance). In addition to biomarker testing to discover your baseline, most offer consultations, wearable data integration, AI-powered insights, and customized health plans based on your results. Companies that fall in this category include Cenegenics, Superpower, Function Health, and Outlive Biology.

If the idea of ordering these tests yourself interests you, or you want to be up to speed on which tests to speak about with your functional medicine practitioner, here are some of the most common to consider:

### *Inflammatory and/or Immune System Markers*

- High-Sensitive CRO (hs-CRP)
- ESR (Sed Rate)
- Systemic Immune-Inflammation Index (SII)
- Systemic Inflammation Response Index (SIRI)
- Ferritin-to-Albumin Ratio (FAR)
- dsDNA Antibody
- CCP Antibody
- Rheumatoid Factor
- ANA (Antinuclear Antibody)
- Thyroid Health Biomarkers
- T3 Uptake
- Free T4 Index
- Thyroxine (T4), Total
- Thyroid Stimulating Hormone (TSH)
- Triiodothyronine (T3), Free

- Thyroid Peroxidase Antibodies (TPO)
- Thyroglobulin Antibodies
- Sex Hormones Biomarkers
- Testosterone, Total
- Sex Hormone Binding Globulin (SHBG)
- Testosterone, Bioavailable
- Testosterone, Free
- Estradiol
- Progesterone
- Follicle Stimulating Hormone (FSH)
- DHEA Sulfate
- Prolactin
- PSA, Prostate Specific Antigen, Free
- Metabolic Health Biomarkers
- Glucose
- Hemoglobin A1c
- Insulin
- Corrected Calcium
- Uric Acid
- Triglyceride- Glucose Index
- Additional Health Biomarkers
- Vitamin B12
- Vitamin D, 25-Hydroxy
- Folate
- MMA, Methylmalonic Acid
- Homocysteine
- Complete Kidney Panel
- Cortisol
- Iron Saturation

- Ferritin
- Total Iron Binding Capacity

### *Medical-Grade Supplementation to Discuss with Your Functional Medicine Doctor or Research on Your Own:*

Depending on your blood and/or saliva results, plus discoveries you made in Tier 1 regarding allergies and microbiome deficiencies, you can use all of that data plus current symptoms that are bothersome and work with your practitioner in choosing medical-grade supplements. Some of the most popular supplements used in the functional medicine world when it comes to chronic illness revolve around:

1. **Reducing overall inflammation/pain**: Medical-grade functional medicine supplements to help decrease inflammation come in a variety of formulas from powders, shakes, capsules, liquid, and even gummies. They typically include a variety of powerful botanical extracts and nutrients such as turmeric and black pepper, ginger, omega-3 fatty acids, boswellia, quercetin, green tea extracts, resveratrol, marine lipid concentrates, and vitamin C.
2. **Supporting adrenal health:** Functional medicine adrenal health and support supplements typically contain adaptogenic herbs, B-complex, vitamin C, and key minerals which work together to help the body manage stress and support the adrenal glands. Adaptogenic herbs are often main ingredients in these formulas, typically derived from herbs and mushrooms, that help the body adapt to mental and physical stress by modulating the stress response. Common ingredients you will see in these formulations include ashwagandha,

rhodiola, holy basil, licorice root, Siberian ginseng, Chinese yam, rehmannia, zinc, magnesium, B vitamins (typically B5, B6, B12 and folate, which are critical when the body is experiencing long-term stressors), and L-theanine.

3. **Reducing brain fog and increasing mental clarity:** Brain fog and reduced clarity can be an ongoing struggle when someone is living with a chronic illness and have a direct effect on mental acuity and performance levels. Functional medicine supplements targeting these issues usually work to reduce inflammation, support neurotransmitter production, improve circulation, and balance the stress response. You will typically find ingredients such as EPA, DHA, B vitamins, magnesium, turmeric, ashwagandha, ginkgo biloba, lion's mane mushrooms, L-theanine, NAC—N-acetyl cysteine, ALCAR—acetyl-L-carnitine, and vitamin D in many formulations.
4. **Restoring gut health on a deeper level:** Since 70 to 80 percent of our immune system resides in our gut, this is usually a key area many functional medicine practitioners like to address with their patients. There are many stronger, more comprehensive gut formulations to help those with severe gut disorders who haven't seen noticeable improvement through dietary changes or pre/pro/postbiotic introduction discussed in Tier 1. More advanced gut health supplementation options include powders/shakes (perfect for individuals having a difficult time digesting solid foods), capsules, chewables, and tinctures. Some of the most common functional medicine gut repair ingredients include digestive enzymes, rosemary, quercetin MCTs, prebiotics/fiber, L-glutamine, slippery

elm bark, aloe vera, zinc, turmeric, and hops. Powders/meal shakes are typically found in vegan pea or rice protein blends that are dairy and gluten free. These ingredients target repair of the gut lining, reduce inflammation of the gut, and help balance the microbe population.

5. **Increasing energy levels**: Another key area functional medicine practitioners look at is energy levels and if they are lacking, target either cellular energy production (ATP), improving mitochondrial function, reducing stress or addressing nutrient deficiencies (addressing adrenal health, discussed above, can also be an issue if energy levels are low). Common ingredients used in functional medicine formulations include B vitamins, iron, vitamin D, magnesium, ginseng, maca, L-carnitine, taurine, rhodiola rosea, ashwagandha, CoQ10, ALA, creatine, green tea extract and L-theanine.
6. **Decreasing allergic responses and histamine**: When chronic illness is present, functional medicine practitioners often explore mast cell and histamine imbalances as potential culprits behind ongoing issues such as hives, itching, flushing, swelling, sinus congestion, digestive upset, and even migraines or unexplained fatigue. When OTC antihistamines aren't enough or create more side effects than solutions, targeted supplementation may offer some relief by helping the body naturally stabilize histamine levels and calm inflammation. Some of the most common ingredients used in formulations include quercetin, a plant flavonoid known for its antioxidant and mast cell–stabilizing properties, and bromelain, an enzyme derived from pineapple that enhances

absorption and supports healthy inflammatory response. Others include vitamin C, stinging nettle leaf, DAO (diamine oxidase) to help break down histamine in food, luteolin, and zinc, which plays a role in immune modulation. I am a big believer in these ingredients and have used them with great success to lessen my allergic responses.

### A Note Before You Dive Into the Powder

The ingredients listed above are some of the most commonly used heavy hitters in the world of medical-grade supplementation—but they're not the only players on the field. These are just the tip of the iceberg, friend. Depending on your test results, symptoms, sensitivities, and your short- or long-term health goals, your supplement protocol may include additional vitamins, minerals, herbs, amino acids, or therapeutic compounds tailored to your body's needs.

That's why it's always wise to partner with a practitioner, coach, or provider who truly understands how these supplements interact with existing conditions, meds, and allergies. Functional medicine formulas aren't your average drugstore vitamins—they're potent, precision-formulated, and in many cases, designed to do the heavy lifting where your body needs it most.

I say this from personal experience: I could actually *feel* the difference within days of starting my first functional medicine protocol—and believe me, I'd never said that about a chalky multivitamin from the drugstore shelf. Over time, the right supplements helped me reclaim energy, stabilize my symptoms, get out of a wheelchair for good, and even reduce my pharma med list from twelve down to four. That's the kind of support these tools can offer when used wisely and intentionally.

## *Deeper Herbology for Chronic Inflammation and Immune Support*

Now it's time to dig into the apothecary section of Tier 2, where we will take a deeper look at some bold, bitter, brain-calming, and bug-busting botanicals that some people with chronic illness swear by. Adding in potent herbs may help tackle a variety of symptoms from brain fog and joint pain to lowering viral loads and regulating the vagal nerve. Think of this section as your leafy, rooty treasure map, sans magic wand, but just as magical. Whether you decide to work with a trained herbalist in your area or remotely, a Chinese medicine specialist, or a functional medicine practitioner that is well-researched in this area, here are some of the most applauded herbs in the chronic illness community:

**Nettle (Urtica dioica)**—Don't let the sting of nettle's fresh leaves scare you away. When its leaves are cooked and prepared properly, this little herb is highly regarded because of its antihistamine effects. Loved by many allergy sufferers, nettle is also known for its ability to reduce inflammation and act as a diuretic.[1] It's most commonly consumed as a tea, tincture, or in pill form, but should not be used in people taking blood thinners or diuretics, or those that have blood pressure issues.

**Holy Basil (Ocimum sanctum, Tulsi)**—Nicknamed "The Incomparable One" because of its wide-reaching benefits, holy basil is a powerful herb that has adaptogenic, anti-inflammatory, antioxidant, and stress-relieving qualities.[2] In chronic illness patients, holy basil is often used to help decrease inflammation, reduce pain and swelling, lower cortisol levels, ease anxiety, improve the body's overall immune response, and has antimicrobial effects.[3] It should not be taken by pregnant or nursing women, those on diabetes medication or blood thinners, or before surgery.

**Astragalus (Astragalus membranaceus, Huáng Qí)**—Astragalus is revered in Traditional Chinese Medicine as one of the best immune-boosting herbs that may also reduce inflammation and help in fighting infections. The National Institute of Health studies indicate it can help regulate overactive immune/inflammatory responses.[4] Additionally, other trials indicate it can help with fatigue in chronic fatigue syndrome and is often used in long-haul COVID protocols.[5] It is taken via capsules, powder, tinctures, or as a tea. This powerful herb should not be taken in combination with lithium, blood pressure medications, immunosuppressants, and blood thinners.

**Licorice Root (Glycyrrhiza glabra)**—One of my top two favorite herbs, this versatile little gem is notable for its adrenal supporting, anti-inflammatory and antiviral effects. It is believed to help inhibit the replication of certain viruses (including coronaviruses), soothe mouth sores, help support adrenal glands and energy levels, and suppress inflammatory mediators.[6] You can find it in mouth rinses, body cream, tinctures, capsules, and teas. Licorice root should not be used by pregnant/nursing women or those with low potassium levels, heart/kidney/liver diseases, or taking certain medications.

**Ashwagandha (Withania somnifera)**—My other beloved herb, ashwagandha is considered the top tier adaptogenic herb because of how it helps the body cope with stress, immune challenges, and loves to love on your stressed-out adrenal glands. Research shows it has an anti-inflammatory effect in the body, and is helpful for conditions like arthritis and neuroinflammatory issues.[7] Additional research shows ashwagandha reduces elevated cortisol and has a calming effect on insomnia and anxiety often experienced by those with chronic illness.[8] It is most commonly found in capsule, pill, or liquid form and should not be used by those with thyroid conditions, hormone-sensitive cancers, certain autoimmune diseases, or pregnant/nursing women.

Always work with a trained practitioner or clinical herbalist when dabbling in plant medicine—herbs may be natural, but they are far from mild-mannered. These little powerhouses can soothe inflammation, boost immunity, and ease pain, but even small amounts can be potent and they can also interact with medications faster than you can say "whoops."

Now, here's a twist I didn't see coming: My first introduction to herbs didn't happen in a health food aisle, at an herbalist's office, or an apothecary—it happened in my rheumatologist's office. Crazy, right? Yep, the very place most people associate with prescription pads and lab coats. I spotted a magazine in the waiting room with an ad for an herbal pain formula called Zyflamend, casually ripped it out (sorry, not sorry), and brought it in to show my doc and save for later. To my surprise, she told me she had several patients who swore by it—and since I wasn't on any heavy-duty immunosuppressants at the time, we gave it the green light to test it out. That blend turned out to be one of the most helpful herbal tools in my rotation, and it's still in my toolbox today for flare-y seasons when I need a little extra leafy love. Funny when life throws you an unexpected but helpful curveball!

### *Exploring Environmental Toxins*

Time for a little pivot—because if you're on a mission to uncover what's stirring the pot in your symptom stew, you've got to look beyond the usual suspects. Just like we run allergy panels and blood tests to figure out what our body is reacting to, it's equally important to ask: Could environmental toxins be silently crashing the party and dysregulating the immune system?[9] Two of the biggest gatecrashers are mold and heavy metals.

These toxin troublemakers don't usually show up waving red flags or shouting, "Hey, I'm the problem!" like a dramatic food allergy might. Nope, they prefer slowly sabotaging your gut health, hormones, immune function, and energy reserves like silent little wrecking balls. And over time? Boom: inflammation, fatigue, joint pain, and yes, they may even fan the flames of autoimmune illness. Delightful, right? But don't worry, we've got ways to track them down.

And here's the kicker with environmental toxins: If you haven't had some dramatic, Hollywood-level exposure, like falling into a vat of mercury or living within a mushroom farm, most traditional doctors will tell you that you don't need to test for them. But in functional medicine, these subtle saboteurs are very much on the radar. Practitioners in this space understand that chronic, low-level exposure—say, from an old moldy apartment or a mouth full of metal fillings—can quietly wreak havoc over time in certain individuals. And spoiler alert: These toxins don't just pack up and leave on their own eventually. They like to settle in and overstay their welcome.

First, let's talk about mold. Mold exposure doesn't just cause a sniffle or two; it can mess with nearly every system in your body. We're talking brain fog, relentless fatigue, chronic sinus infections, congestion that never quits, asthma-like wheezing, hives, weird chemical sensitivities, autoimmune flares . . . it's basically the worst Airbnb guest your immune system never asked for.

Then there are heavy metals, charming characters like mercury, lead, cadmium, and arsenic, which like to interfere with your nervous system and cellular function. Symptoms often creep up slowly: metallic taste in your mouth, unexplained fatigue, tremors, digestive issues, brain fog, and that delightful pins-and-needles feeling in your hands or feet.

But here's the good news: You don't have to sit around guessing anymore like sufferers did decades ago. We live in a time where testing has finally caught up to our symptoms. You can now order noninvasive at-home urine mycotoxin panels to see if your body's hoarding mold toxins or swab and dust tests to check if your living space is the problem. And when it comes to metals? Hair and blood analysis can give you a much-needed window into your toxic load. In other words, you're not imagining the correlation between possible exposure and strange, erratic symptoms—and now, you can prove it.

When testing for mold or heavy metals, the tools are quite different depending on whether you're testing your body or your environment. For testing your body, ask your functional medicine practitioners about completing a urine mycotoxin tests (like RealTime Labs or Great Plains/ Mosaic Diagnostics) to detect mold toxins, and doing a hair or blood mineral analysis from Doctor's Data or Trace Elements Inc. to check for heavy metals like mercury, lead, or arsenic. If you believe mold might be present in your home or apartment, some of the most popular mold test kits include My Mold Detective, EnviroBiomics ERMI tests, and ImmunoLytics, which can test both surface and air, depending on the test. Body testing tells you what's *inside* you; environmental testing tells you what you're *being exposed to*, and both are crucial!

### *Conducting a Clean Sweep of Other Environmental Toxins*

I felt the chemical cocktail we slather on ourselves daily deserved its own stage. It's serious and you are likely to put these chemicals on or in your body each and every day. I am talking about petrochemicals, phthalates, parabens, formaldehyde releasers, and endocrine disruptors. These are most often found in shampoos and conditioners, body lotions, skin care, makeup, hair color, cleansers, toothpaste, perfumes, and hair products.

And men, you aren't as far removed from these chemicals as you may think you are, as they are also found in beard and men's hair products, colognes, and even fitness supplements. But women take on the greatest hazard from these chemical cocktails, as we use over 160 of these chemicals each and every day on average.[10] A little beachy-smelly spritz here, some blush and mascara there, a little dry shampoo here, and dab of lipstick there. What is the point of doing so much work in the areas of food, supplementation, and nervous system retraining, if we are only going to turn around the same day and overload our body with chemicals it can't process?

So, if you are stuck in cycles of fatigue, inflammation, histamine overload, or good old mysterious symptoms, you may be literally overlooking the daily invaders that are keeping your entire body on defense mode.

These types of chemicals not only destroy your hormones, they wreck your immune system, burden your liver, and disrupt your nervous system. You might be asking why people with chronic illness need to take these types of chemicals very seriously. Here's a few things to consider regarding how these chemicals affect the body:

- **Products made with parabens and phthalates** are known endocrine disruptors, which can block or mimic natural hormones in the body. When these chemicals interfere with our natural state, symptoms like fertility issues, irregular periods, weight gain, or even thyroid dysfunction can occur.

- **Shampoo, clothing, detergent, lipstick** and even some medicines contain petrochemicals like toluene and benzene derivatives. These known neurotoxins literally destroy your central nervous system, slowly at first and accumulate over time, leaving a trail of potential symptoms behind such as dizziness, anxiety, and brain fog.
- **Immune agitating chemicals**, such as synthetic fragrance, preservatives, triclosan, and formaldehyde to name a few, act like little alarm bells for your immune system, liberating histamine responses and increasing inflammation. These chemicals are most often found in your cosmetics, nail polish, food colorings, soaps, lotions, and shampoos and can exacerbate allergy, eczema, rhinitis and asthma.
- **Liver stressing chemicals**, such as PFAs, PCE and VOCs, slow down detoxing pathways in our liver—the body's ultimate filter—and can cause a variety of issues such as breakouts, poor digestion, sluggishness and sensitivities to chemicals and medications. These chemicals are found in stain-resistant fabrics (think your furniture), nonstick pans, microwave popcorn bags, and certain clothing.

What can we do to combat this daily chemical assault? A chemical cleanse doesn't have to mean trashing everything at once and running barefoot into a field of organic lavender unless that's your vibe, in which case—I salute you and I'd totally join you. But a more realistic, sustainable approach is this: As each personal care product runs out, swap it for a cleaner alternative. Use apps like Think Dirty, Yuka, or EWG's Skin Deep to scan ingredients for body products, makeup, and even food choices so you become more informed over time. Stick to brands that disclose full ingredient lists, and watch out for two of the most vague culprits:

"Fragrance"—An ambiguous label ingredient that is most often a combination of synthetic chemicals.[11]

"Natural flavors"—Another nebulous label ingredient that can be defined as a complex combination of solvents, chemicals, and preservatives derived from a natural source but heavily processed.[12]

When curating a long-term lifestyle with lower amounts of chemical cocktails, start with what covers the most real estate: think body lotion, shampoo, facial moisturizer, deodorant, and makeup if you wear it daily. These are the big hitters. From there, move into nail polish, sunscreen, and even laundry detergent, dish soap, and hand soap—because what touches your skin matters.

Physical symptoms you might see improve over time as you product detox include:

- Hormonal acne
- Migraines or brain fog
- Histamine flares
- Itchy, rashy skin
- Worsening allergies or asthma
- Endocrine imbalances (like thyroid or cortisol dysregulation)

This step of Tier 2 is important because you're creating an environment that's less hostile to your body. And when your system isn't under chemical siege from morning to evening, it can shift resources back toward repair, resilience, and—dare we say it—actual healing.

### *Let's Talk About Lymph, Baby*

Lymph is the unsung hero of your immune system and one of the most underappreciated fluids sloshing around in your body every day. Your lymphatic system is basically the body's drainage system, sweeping up toxins, waste, excess fluids, and even cellular debris like it's tidying up after a spring-break college party.[13] This clear-to-white fluid also transports infection-fighting white blood cells, making it a major player in immune support and inflammation control. But here's the catch: Unlike your blood, which gets pumped around by your heart, lymph doesn't have its own "pump" per se. It relies on muscle movement, deep breathing, staying hydrated, exercising regularly and even wearing compression garments in some instances.

It can also be moved around with some outside encouragement—enter lymphatic drainage massage. This type of massage is a gentle, rhythmic technique that helps stimulate the movement of lymph so it can drain properly through your lymph nodes (your body's detox command centers). We aren't talking about deep-tissue, knuckles-pressed-in-your-back kind of work. Lymph work is light, precise, and surprisingly relaxing.

For people with chronic illness, where inflammation is already high and detox pathways are often sluggish, lymph massage can be a game changer. In time you'll notice less puffiness, increased energy, fewer headaches, and improved immune resilience. It can also help move out lingering toxins, especially if you're detoxing from mold, metals, or the petrochemicals we just talked about.

Why does lymph get sluggish in the first place? Chronic illness often brings fatigue, low mobility, and a stressed-out nervous system—all stop signs which basically slow lymph flow to a crawl. Add in dehydration, gut issues, or a sluggish liver, and your drainage system can get as backed up as a traffic jam in rush hour.

How do you know if your lymph isn't draining well? Look out for signs like unexplained swelling, especially in hands, feet, or under your eyes, ongoing battles against infections, brain fog, fatigue, or even skin breakouts. If you're waking up feeling as swollen as the Michelin Man, your lymph may be asking for help.

You can work with a trained lymphatic massage therapist (bonus points if they have experience with chronic illness) or try some DIY lymph massage at home. Lymphatic massage always begins around the neck/collarbone area and then moves to other areas of the body.[14] Other ways to increase movement of lymph that can be performed at home include: dry brushing, rebounding on a mini trampoline (if tolerated), and meeting your daily fluid intake like it's your part-time job. The goal? Keep things flowing—literally—so your body has a fighting chance to heal and detox. Quick disclaimer though on lymph massage, while this technique can have numerous health advantages, it is contraindicated in anyone with blood clots, cellulitis, heart disease, and kidney disease.

### Adding On a Centuries Old Drainage Method

If lymphatic drainage got your attention and you are starting to get the hang of the entire "drain your lymph" thing (love that for you), then guess what? There is another ancient therapy that deserves a seat at the table, at least for a conversation: wet cupping. Wet cupping has been practiced for centuries across many cultures, such as Chinese and Greek traditional medicine, but has deep roots in Arab medicine. Research shows it can specifically help with rheumatic conditions, sluggish draining, and particularly pain. In fact, as the National Institute of Health states, that pain is the main reason people seek alternative and complementary therapies, it shows there is increasing evidence that this type of cupping can help decrease several types of pain.[15] And speaking of pain, numerous studies have stated wet cupping as a beneficial therapy for those with fibromyalgia pain.[16]

While dry cupping uses suction alone, wet cupping combines suction with tiny skin incisions to draw out a small amount of blood and interstitial fluid. And while it may sound like medieval bloodletting, it's done in a controlled, hygienic setting by a trained practitioner—and many folks with chronic inflammation and pain swear by it.

How does wet cupping relieve these types of symptoms? Think of wet cupping as your lymphatic system's jumpstart cable. When done correctly, it:

- **Stimulates stagnant fluid movement**, which is critical if your lymph is as sluggish as you feel.
- **Supports detox pathways**, helping clear out inflammatory byproducts or what practitioners call "stuck blood."
- **Relieves pain and pressure**, especially in areas where circulation is compromised.
- **May help modulate immune responses**, which is key in autoimmunity or chronic infection.

While lymph massage gently nudges your body to move fluid, wet cupping creates a more forceful "vacuum and release" effect. Think of it as calling in a pressure washer for your fascia and capillaries. They're different tools for the same sluggish system. And no, you don't need to choose one over the other—many people alternate them depending on what their body needs in that season.

But a few caveats: Wet cupping isn't a fit for everyone. And it is absolutely not something you are going to perform at home on yourself. If you're dealing with blood clotting disorders, have very low immune function, anemia, are on blood thinners, or have super-sensitive/thin skin, this might not be your go-to therapy. Always work with a licensed or highly trained practitioner that is experienced in your diagnosis and the symptoms you are experiencing.

## Tier 2 Wrap-Up: Look at You Grow

Phew. Can you believe we've made it to the end of Tier 2? If Tier 1 was all about putting down roots, this phase was where the real sprouting happened. And if your brain is feeling slightly overloaded from all the detox tools, testing options, and supplement protocols—that's totally normal. Take a breath. Take stock. You've experienced a lot of trial and error over these two tiers.

You've explored an entire ecosystem of healing beyond pharmaceuticals: deeper allergy testing, blood biomarkers, functional medicine, medical-grade supplementation, adrenal and inflammation support, mold and metal exposure, lymph drainage, acupuncture, petrochemical purging, and more. Honestly, it's enough to make a conventional doctor's stethoscope spin right off their shoulders.

Whether you've tackled these over a few focused months or taken a scenic, year-long stroll through this garden of healing, *please* take a moment to acknowledge yourself. You're doing the work. You're introducing your body to life-changing options. You're starting to see what helps your body bloom.

So, before we move into Tier 3—our final tier—I want you to check in with yourself. Grab a notebook and dig into these questions:

- Which new therapies or protocols did I try in Tier 2?
- What surprised me the most about how my body responded?

- Were there any clear wins—shifts in energy, fewer flares, better digestion, less inflammation?
- Which tools felt supportive enough to earn a spot in my "master gardener" toolbox?
- Did anything feel like too much, too soon? (No shame, here; timing is everything)
- Are there areas I want to revisit or dig deeper into later with more support?
- What felt empowering about experimenting outside the standard medical model?
- What am I most proud of from this tier? (Celebrate it, even if it's "I remembered to take my supplements three days in a row.")
- Am I ready for Tier 3, or do I need more time here to gather data and feel steady?

# CHAPTER 12

# THE ROOT & BLOOM PROTOCOL TIER 3: BLOOM

If you've made it this far, you're not just surviving chronic illness, you are doing the experimentations and actively rewriting your healing story. You've dug into your roots, nurtured your body through the slow-and-steady Grow phase, and now it's time to *Bloom.*

This tier is all about expanding your capacity, widening the lanes of energy, resilience, and restoration you've been slowly building. We're talking advanced tools now that help speed recovery and support deeper repair: IV nutrition, infrared saunas, hydrotherapy, cryo- and hyperbaric chambers, and even a surprise "functional-pharma" twist. You've already done the heavy lifting of figuring out what helps you feel better, now we're layering in the heavy equipment.

Welcome to your next level.

## Finding Healing in the Most Unexpected Places

Over a decade ago, I landed in one of my favorite cities—Chicago—for a week-long advocacy summit and focus groups. And let's just say

. . . I was already running on fumes as I embarked. Coming off the tail end of a flare, my body hit the "nope" button by day two. Five more days to go and then a nine-hour drive home? Absolutely not. I needed backup, quick, or I knew a hospital visit was most likely in my immediate future.

So off I went to the local Whole Foods to grab some green juice, and while there, a local friend texted me a tip that would unexpectedly add yet another level to my healing journey: "You need to check out the IV drip bar down the street. The Myers Cocktails I've been getting have been lifesavers during some of my worst Lyme days." Intrigued, and frankly desperate—I decided to go.

Back then, IV clinics weren't exactly on every corner, so walking into one felt like stepping into a futuristic wellness Disneyland. There was an actual menu of vitamin and nutrient "cocktails," each tailored to different health issues: autoimmune, cancer, inflammation, fatigue, energy, you name it. And yes, I wanted to try them *all.* But . . . I was hesitant.

Now, I won't lie: I am absolutely a chicken when it comes to trying new things. But I also live by the motto "do it scared"—because otherwise, I'll overthink it until I've talked myself right back into bed. I knew if I didn't try something, anything, I was headed straight for another flare and wouldn't be able to finish the advocacy conference. So, I sat with the nurse practitioner, went down a lengthy list of my conditions, symptoms, allergies and current ailments, rolled up my sleeve and took the plunge. And that moment kicked off my ongoing love affair with IV nutrition therapy, which, lucky for all of us, is now *way* more accessible than it used to be and popping up in cities across the world.

### *IV Therapy 101*

Also called intravenous micronutrient therapy, IV nutrition therapy provides various cocktails of minerals, vitamins, amino acids, antioxidants, and fluids that rush straight into your bloodstream: meaning it gets to work right away because it bypasses the digestive tract entirely. Though it has been around much longer, it became more popular in functional medicine and integrative clinics in the early 2000s. Depending on the clinic, you'll be met with "cocktails" of certain recipes that are made specifically for symptoms found in autoimmune diseases, cancer, long-haul COVID, dehydration, inflammation, chronic pain, and more.

One of the most popular "cocktails" is the Myers' Cocktail, created and first administered by Dr. John Myers in the 1970s, is popular in Lyme circles, and was originally used for chronic fatigue, asthma, and headaches.[1] Today, cocktails include ingredients such as vitamin C, vitamin B, magnesium, glutathione, and trace minerals, to name a few. Specific combinations can be made depending on what symptoms are most bothersome to you, and can help reduce inflammation and pain, boost energy, hydrate, and also help detox.

Today, most IV nutrition drips are given in an IV bar or functional medicine clinic under medical supervision. A trained and licensed medical professional has to deliver the infusion, one who understands your medical history, current medications, allergies, etc. IV infusions may not be right for you if you deal with heart issues, electrolyte imbalances, or kidney conditions.

While many report an almost-instant perk in energy and increased feeling of well-being, I can tell you I felt a major shift within an hour of getting my very first infusion. It worked so well, I got another before I left Chicago and they have been a part of my healing regimen ever since.

### ***Now Let's Go Back in Time. . . . Halotherapy***

Shortly after my love affair with IV nutrition began, I was introduced to another healing therapy that immediately was a forever addition to my "master toolbox." While my dad struggled with late-stage cancer complications, a dear friend of his opened up an authentic salt cave just outside of New York City in Port Washington. Ok, if you are thinking, *this is way too Woo, Woo, Marisa*, just stay with me for a second. You just might be surprised to learn that salt caves (also known as Halotherapy) have been around for centuries and have a wide variety of benefits. Salt caves originated in Eastern Europe (we see you, Poland!), with salt therapy unexpectedly originating at the renowned Wieliczka Salt Mine. Dr. Feliks Boczkowski observed in the early nineteenth-century that salt miners had little to no respiratory issues or conditions and founded the first "salt cave" underground health facility serving people with asthma and allergies at this mine.

Halotherapy involves sitting in a room that has a halogenerator machine dispersing micro-particles of pharmaceutical grade pure sodium chloride (salt) which mimics natural salt caves. Beneficial effects of salt caves[2] include reducing inflammation, clearing airways, improving respiratory conditions, and lung function in asthma, emphysema, COPD (even the NIH backs this up) improving allergies, and helping the body detox. The incredibly fine salt particles also release negative ions, which are believed to benefit cells, while mucus and inflammation in the lungs and skin are also cleared due to the natural antiseptic properties in salt. To enhance the experience, many salt caves have the floors and walls covered in Himalayan salt.

An added bonus of many of today's salt caves are that they are dimly lit, relaxing, cooler in temperature, and an ideal, quiet place to not only relax in silence but enjoy healing benefits as you do it. When

I am not writing or road-tripping, you can often find me in a salt cave with my headphones, chill play list, and fluffy blanket.

### *Let's Talk Regenerative: Hyperbaric Oxygen Therapy*

In the spirit of growing and blooming, let's take a quick look at another regenerative healing modality: Hyperbaric Oxygen Therapy (HBOT). Ready for a plot twist? Well, one of the most underrated anti-inflammatory powerhouses for issues like chronic pain, fibromyalgia, and inflammation is . . . good old oxygen![3] HBOT involves breathing 100 percent pure oxygen inside a pressurized chamber. Think Jetson's space pod, where you relax and basically just inhale. The increased pressure inside these pods allows for more oxygen to dissolve into your blood plasma. The result? It can reach areas of inflamed or damaged tissues that are desperately seeking more oxygen in order to heal.

HBOT is quite popular in Western medicine when it comes to wound healing and traumatic brain injuries, but it's become increasingly sought-after in cases of mold illness, long-haul COVID, autoimmune diseases, Lyme, and more. The logic around this surge? Having more oxygen available equals reduced inflammation, greater tissue repair, immune modulation, and greater support of the mitochondria. Multiple sessions are typically required and are available at hospitals, wellness clinics, and some functional medicine wellness labs. And, depending on your condition, insurance might pick up the tab.

While a game changer for many, there are some caveats around HBOT to be aware of: It can be costly, and it is not for the claustrophobic. Also, if you have COPD or asthma, untreated collapsed lung, high fever/flu, recent ear surgery or ear injury, you will want to skip this protocol.

### *Back to the Basics: Hydrotherapy*

Long before IV nutrition clinics and HBOT wellness spots popped up in almost every town, there was good old-fashioned water. And with plenty of research confirming the use of hot and cold water exposure as beneficial for rheumatic diseases,[4] fibromyalgia,[5] and inflammatory issues, Hydrotherapy has reentered the chat. Hydrotherapy harnesses water's temperature, pressure, and movement to stimulate the body's healing response. Think warm soaks, cold plunges, contrast showers, and pulsing therapeutic jets that know exactly where tension lives in the body. You may be calling it old-school, but in the best, most effective way.

You might be wondering, *what is actually happening when you take part in a hydrotherapy session*? Alternating hot and cold exposure helps expand and constrict your blood vessels, which then improves circulation, helps tissues flush out waste, decreases inflammation, and circling back to earlier, helps crack a whip, so to speak, on that sluggish lymph—which we know could definitely use a nudge if you're chronically ill.

Warm water relaxes tight muscles and stimulates parasympathetic (rest-and-digest) nervous system responses, while cold water tones the vascular system, supports detox, and reduces swelling. When you combine the two together in one session, known as contrast hydrotherapy, they create a kind of internal workout for your circulation and immune system.

And here's the best part: You can actually begin this type of therapy in your very own bathroom. Contrast showers can be done right at home (hot water for three minutes, cold blast for thirty seconds, repeat), and if you aren't ready to start full body right now, even foot soaks with alternating temps can promote systemic effects. Want to take hydrotherapy to the next level? Physical therapists and many wellness centers offer water-based rehab sessions, and therapeutic spas often include hydrotherapy in their chronic illness care menus.

And similar to other therapies out there (just give Gerson therapy a Google), Europe's been onto hydrotherapy forever. In fact, providers in Germany regularly prescribe spa therapy, and the US is slowly catching up.[6] Some insurance plans may cover hydro-based PT sessions under rehabilitation if you have a documented condition. But if taking on an outside hydrotherapy expense is not in the cards at the moment, just give your bathtub or shower time a promotion. Contraindications for hydrotherapy include people with uncontrolled blood pressure, uncontrolled heart conditions, open wounds, fear of water, and skin infections.

### *You Bloomed, Baby*

Phew. You made it through Tier 3! And, if you're still here with highlighters in hand, covered in Post-it notes, or surrounded by data-filled notebooks, let me just say: You're a legend. We've just covered quite an exhaustive list to get you started on your healing path—and that's the condensed version (honestly, we'd need another volume). But what you have within these pages and in your notes and experiences is a comprehensive roadmap to get started in reclaiming your energy, easing your symptoms, and building a life that actually supports your body.

The Root and Bloom Protocol is designed to be layered and lived. It is rooted in experimentation, not rushed through. And as you have probably come to realize along the way, healing isn't linear. You may bounce between tiers at times. Maybe you revisit Tier 1 to update your allergy testing and see if sensitivities have calmed down, or you want to see what changes have occurred in your microbiome. Or maybe you hit pause on a therapy from Tier 2 and circle back once you're in a more stable place. That's not failure, that's intelligent healing. It's getting to know your body intimately all over again and listening when your body says, "I'm ready to try this now," or "This is too much for me in this season."

And now, as a wrap up for the protocol, I want to share with you the two sub tiers I mentioned at the start of this protocol: a deeper dive into the spiritual, energetic, and emotional sides of healing that many people never even think to touch. Because we're not just living in the physical realm. We are triune beings—mind, body, and spirit—and healing one layer without acknowledging the others will only get you halfway home.

These upcoming sections are about nourishment beyond nutrients. They're about uncovering the emotional patterns, energetic wounds, and nervous system overloads that so often sit at the root of disease.

When you're ready to step into those sub tiers, take your time. Read with curiosity, not pressure. Explore what resonates now and shelve what doesn't for later. Add in throughout Tier 1 to Tier 3 when you feel comfortable building another layer.

Before you move on, take a moment to check in with yourself post–Tier 3 experimentation. These questions can help solidify what's going in your Master Gardener Toolbox as you move forward:

Reflection Questions:

1. Which therapies or protocols in Tier 3 gave you the biggest return in energy, symptom relief, or overall wellness?
2. Are there treatments you were initially unsure about that ended up surprising you in a good way?

3. Were there any therapies that didn't resonate or caused side effects—and what did they teach you about your body's needs?
4. What's one to two tools from each tier you can commit to continuing in your regular routine?
5. Do you feel more connected to your body than when you started this journey?
6. Are there practitioners, communities, or resources you want to keep in your long-term support circle?
7. What does "healing" look like to you *now* compared to when you first started?
8. Are there symptoms you haven't revisited in a while that may need updated testing or approaches?
9. What do you feel most hopeful about right now in terms of your health?

So, take a breath—a big, proud, possibly tear-filled breath. You've done the work. You dug deep into the roots, watered what was dry, cleared what no longer served, and little by little, started growing and reaching toward the light.

This isn't just symptom-chasing anymore—this is you reclaiming agency over your health and crafting a life that fits *your* body. And now? You're blooming—not perfectly, not all at once, but boldly and in your own time. That's not just healing. That is transformation. As the years go by, you will undoubtedly learn about and try different therapies and approaches. You will see even further results, and you will be grateful that you never gave up on yourself. And don't forget, I'm at the sidelines with my poms-poms, rooting for you. Pun intended!

# CHAPTER 13

# THE ROOT & BLOOM PROTOCOL: SUB TIERS

Before we go any further, green juice in hand, amiga to amiga, I need to tell you something important—and yes, it's in all caps: THE SUB TIERS DO NOT GO LAST. These are the deeply human, soul-stretching, often-ignored pieces of healing that can shift the whole healing game—and they deserve their own proper introduction.

You'll pull practices from the two sub tiers into your main tiers when your body, your spirit, or your gut instinct says, *Now. I'm ready for this part.* Whether it's acupuncture and massage, or art therapy and prayer, or even spiritual inquiry, the sub tiers are all about layering in healing that nourishes your *whole* self.

And that's where we get into the good stuff. Because you, my friend, are not just a bundle of symptoms walking around in a body. You're a triune being—body, mind, and spirit—and real healing happens when all three areas are paid attention to. That's why I talk about therapy as much as ginger. That's why these practices—Bodywork and Mind-Body-Spirit—are not footnotes. They're a coming-home.

Take what speaks to you. What your mind lingers on after you turn the page. Try what feels safe. Leave what doesn't. But know this: You're allowed to go deeper. And you never have to do it all at once. Choose practices from the sub tiers as you work your way through the entire protocol, as your energy grows and your curiosity kicks in.

Ready? Let's go!

## The Bodywork Sub Tier

Truth: As you work through the three main tiers of The Root & Bloom Protocol, there is a lot of *thinking* taking place. Many considerations regarding what your body is ready to take on, and what testing kit, protocol, or supplement you are wanting to try next and then implementing it into your life. Some of those decisions may feel a bit overwhelming or nerve-wracking at times because you are doing something new. And this is where the Bodywork sub tier comes in. It's a sub tier that speaks directly to your body's tissues, muscles, lymph and nervous system. And while relaxation can be found here, it's deeper than that. It's also about regulation—turning the volume down on inflammation, chronic tension, and trauma you may have stored in the body.

Many of the possible practices listed below work specifically on the parasympathetic nervous system (your rest-digest-heal state), which is exactly where long-term healing happens. So, whether you're working with a skilled practitioner in your area or doing some of these practices at home, these are ways to get *in* your body, allow your nervous system to relax, and help it finally feel safe enough to heal.

### *Craniosacral Therapy*

I promise you don't need a neuroscience degree to understand what Craniosacral Therapy means. In fact, it's just a somewhat intimidating word that describes a very gentle bodywork technique that works on the rhythm of the fluid around your brain and spinal cord. Craniosacral massage practitioners use light touch to help release restrictions in that system, supporting the nervous system, reducing pain, and—according to research—easing symptoms like headaches, neck, and back pain, TMJ, fibromyalgia, and even trauma responses.[1] It's subtle but powerful, and sometimes described as "being reset from the inside out."

### *Massage Therapy*

Massage is for more than girlfriends-spa-cations and stress relief (although yes, those are great too). For people with health conditions like autoimmune disease, certain cancers, Parkinson's, fibromyalgia, long-haul COVID, and more, research shows regular massage can improve circulation, reduce inflammation, and calm overworked muscles and nerves.[2] It's also been shown to reduce cortisol and increase serotonin and dopamine—meaning it can *physically shift* your body out of stress mode.[3] Yes, *please.*

### *Acupuncture*

Needles? Yes. Frightening? Not at all (Seriously, they're thinner than a cat's whisker.) Acupuncture taps into the ancient Chinese meridian system to restore flow and balance to the body—think of it as energetic plumbing. Clinical studies show acupuncture helps reduce inflammation, relieve chronic pain, and regulate immune response.[4] It's particularly helpful for autoimmune symptoms and chronic fatigue. Plus, in a serious win for improving mental health, one study of five hundred subjects showed over a 78 percent drop in depression symptoms and a 41 percent decline in anxiety from just six sessions.[5]

Plus, many people find it deeply relaxing, despite the whole needles thing (which are ten times smaller than your average hypodermic needle. You got this!).

### *Reiki*

This energy-based healing method involves no poking, prodding, or manipulation—just hands lightly placed on or above the body to promote energetic alignment and restore balance and flow. Sounds hocusy-pocusy? I suppose it could if you've never tried it. But research shows Reiki can reduce pain, anxiety, and depression in chronically ill patients, by nudging your parasympathetic nervous system into its "rest and restore" mode.[6] Simple Reiki translation: less chaos, more calm. And the best part? The practitioner does all the work. You don't have to *do* anything except show up and soak in the energy, wrapped in a blanket, preferably.

### *Restorative Yoga*

This is not your sweaty power flow or hot yoga retreat. Most chronically ill bodies are a long way from those practices as they begin their healing journey. Please, if you are in a low-functioning season of severe illness, do not jump into those practices which can do more harm than good. Restorative yoga on the other hand, is their cozy cousin—this practice uses props, blankets, and long-held, deeply supported poses to guide your nervous system into chill mode.

This practice was one of my main go-tos early on and is still a part of my life today—though I am known to fall asleep in most of the classes I take (it seriously relaxes you *that much*). Studies show restorative yoga helps regulate cortisol, support digestion, reduce muscle tension, and improve sleep, in addition to lowering inflammation markers.[7] It's the ultimate "do less, heal more" practice, and can also be done in your own home through streaming classes or YouTube if you do not have the energy or wallet to venture out.

### *Grounding Outdoors*

You didn't think I'd give you the condensed version of The Root & Bloom Protocol without actually *rooting yourself*—feet to soil, did you? Grounding might sound a little too crunchy to be legit, but guess what? Science backs it up too. Direct contact with the earth (yes, barefoot in the grass counts) has been shown in studies to reduce inflammation, ease pain, lower stress, and even help you sleep better.[8] The earth's surface carries a subtle negative charge and making contact helps neutralize excess free radicals in the body.

In that connection, your body gets a dose of antioxidant magic—kind of like nature's anti-inflammatory plug-in. So go ahead, kick off your shoes, find a sunny patch of dirt, or even that questionable patch in your backyard, and let the earth do her thing. Your cells, your soul, your entire body will love it.

## The Mind-Body-Spirit Sub Tier

Here we are, friend—the part of your healing journey that tends to raise eyebrows, stir the soul, and sometimes surprise you with just how effective it can be. In this sub tier, I won't be encouraging you to burn sage and chant mantras (unless that's your jam, then by all means go for it). This sub tier revolves more around acknowledging that your mind, emotions, and spirit hold just as much healing power as a fancy supplement or cutting-edge at-home lab panel. And while the physical body has been the star of the show so far, your nervous system, beliefs, emotions, and thoughts are playing major roles behind the curtain.

As a reminder, you don't need to dive into all of these at once (please don't). Just like the first sub tier, the Mind-Body-Spirit tier is something you weave in when you feel safe, curious, or called to. Some of these ideas may intrigue or excite you, and others you may just gloss over. Sprinkle in the ones that interest you during Tier 1 or 2, when your nervous system feels extra fried. Add something new during Tier 3 when your physical symptoms calm down a bit and you're ready to explore the roots. But most importantly, stay open. These practices aren't fluff. In fact, they're backed by science and thousands of years of human experience (all references are available at the end of this book).

### *Art and Music Therapy*

We already covered traditional talk-therapy in multiple areas of this book, but art and music are the therapy outliers I feel we don't hear about often enough and should absolutely be considered. Art therapy is much more than adult coloring books and DIY embroidery patterns. It's a powerful modality that taps into the non-verbal parts of your brain, where trauma, emotions, and stress love to hide.

By engaging in drawing, painting, or sculpting under the guidance of a trained art therapist, patients with chronic illness often find a way to express grief, pain, or frustration they didn't even realize they were carrying. Studies show art therapy reduces anxiety and depression and even improves quality of life for people with chronic conditions like cancer[9] and chronic pain[10] in fibromyalgia and autoimmune disorders.

Art therapy has been my personal go-to for years. If you already follow me online, you have probably seen videos of me painting in my art studio. One thing I have seen time and time again is, I often head into my art room with some wild level of physical pain and emerge hours later with no pain *and* feeling recharged. Plus, art therapy is one of the few "therapies" where you get to be creative, think (or paint) outside of the box (and lines), and get things really messy on purpose.

Music therapy also is an integral piece of the therapy conversation. Whether it's belting Taylor in the car or vibing to a cello suite, music has an uncanny ability to shift your internal world. Music therapy involves listening to, composing, or playing music. It's been studied in cancer patients with evidence showing it helps reduce pain and fatigue, as well as lessening anxiety and depression symptoms.[11] Additional research has shown it reduces cortisol, lowers blood pressure, and boosts mood in patients with chronic pain and chronic disease.[12] For people with chronic illness, it can serve as both emotional release and nervous system regulation. And no, you don't have to be "musical"—your Apple or Spotify playlist totally counts. Though I don't work with a certified music therapist per se, I often find playing my piano at home and listening to healing frequencies (more on this below) through my headphones in a dark room both lessen my perception of physical pain and make me feel happier.

### *Mindfulness Meditation*

Nope, I am not about to tell you to sit cross-legged and think of absolutely nothing for an hour, because, hello, it's completely unrealistic. But I am going to encourage you to take even three to five minutes when you have them to engage in some micro-meditation. Mindfulness meditation can be as simple as noticing your breath for two to three minutes. And the benefits are incredible: Studies show regular meditation reduces inflammation, improves immune response, helps with pain tolerance, and even changes your brain structure in favor of calm and resilience.[13] Whether you prefer a guided app like Calm, Ten Percent Happier (specifically made for skeptics), Headspace, or closing your eyes in a quiet room, this practice rewires your mind-body connection, one breath at a time.

### *Sound Bowl Sessions*

If you've never experienced a sound bath session at your local yoga studio, trust me, you will want to put this on your to-do-list. Sound bowls, often made from quartz or metal, emit frequencies that can synchronize brain waves and guide your body into a more relaxed state. Research on sound-based interventions like binaural beats and vibrational therapy show improvements in mood, anxiety, and even immune response.[14] During a session, you lie down fully clothed while a practitioner gently plays bowls around you.

People often report feeling lighter, calmer, or deeply rested afterward. It's like a vibrational massage for your nervous system. One of my favorite parts of sound bathing is that you can purchase these bowls online, set up a small space, and immerse yourself in your own soothing at-home concert.

### *Prayer*

Whether your faith is rock-solid or more "spiritual-but-questioning," prayer is powerful. Research has shown prayer improves outcomes for those with chronic illness, decreasing anxiety, increasing calmness and helping reduce perceived pain and isolation.[15] Other research shows patients who regularly pray tend to have longer survival rates with chronic conditions over those who do not.[16]

Here is the thing about prayer: There's no "right" way to do it—it's about connection. To something greater. To yourself. To hope. It can look like structured liturgy or a rambling conversation to God or a Higher Power while in the shower. There's no wrong way to talk to the divine.

### *Healing Frequencies*

Last and certainly not least when creating your healing protocol, healing frequencies enter the room. Think of these frequencies as music's more mystical, biohacking cousin. These are specific sound vibrations (like the much-loved 741Hz, 528Hz, or 432Hz) that are believed to interact with your body's natural electromagnetic field and cellular function. Sound a little out there? Stay with me. A quick ten-minute session of these frequencies playing on YouTube while you lie down with your eyes closed may turn you into a believer.

Growing research suggests that certain frequencies may help downshift the nervous system, reduce anxiety, support emotional processing, and even enhance cellular repair.[17] Some practitioners refer to 528Hz as the "miracle tone," as it stems from one of the original Solfeggio frequencies. If you are unfamiliar, Solfeggio frequencies are a set of specific sound tones believed to have unique healing properties. Used for centuries in spiritual and therapeutic practices, each frequency is thought to support different aspects of well-being, like calming the nervous system, easing emotional stress, or even encouraging cellular repair. The 528Hz tone is known for promoting calmness, potential cellular repair, and enhancing feelings of inner peace. Whether you play one of these frequencies during your meditation session discussed above, let it hum in the background while you sleep, or use it to decrease anxiety during a flare, healing frequencies are a gentle, accessible tool with virtually zero downside. Just press play and let all the cells in your body catch the vibe.

## You Did It!

And just like that, we've made it to the end of The Root & Bloom Protocol, tiers, sub tiers and all. As you walk this journey, remember there is no right or wrong way to live out the things I discussed in this protocol. Everyone's path will look different in some way. I encourage you to follow your curiosity and trust your gut. This isn't about sticking to a rigid plan, it's about building a protocol and a life as unique as your symptoms, your story, and your spectacularly resilient self.

I want you to truly, deeply know, what an honor it's been to share the alternative medicine part of my chronic illness journey with you. What you've read throughout this protocol aren't some lofty, untested theories and ideas. It's the condensed, hard-won, soul-poured-out version of everything I've learned from years of experimenting, tweaking, flaring, failing, and rising again. It's how I was able to finally flourish again through many trials and errors and figuring out things along the way!

I didn't come across The Root & Bloom protocol in a textbook.

I've *lived* it. For more than two decades now.

I created it because *I had to*; because I was desperate to get out of a wheelchair, to have more than one "okay" day a week, to simply breathe without pain. I wanted to paint again, take my dog for a walk, and go road-tripping with my husband.

And now? While I still have challenging days (chronic illness doesn't just exactly clock out, as we know), I've reclaimed my ability to travel, work, laugh hard, chase my passions, and feel like an improved and always improving version of myself again. Not the pre-illness version, but a version that's wiser, more compassionate, and pretty badass, if I do say so myself.

So, if you're holding this book and wondering, *Can I really do all of this?*, let me just say this: YES. You already are. You've shown up, you are asking the hard questions, you are believing in your heart that there is something deeper and greater in your future than just illness, and you've dared to hope for something more.

Keep going.

Keep blooming.

You are weaving together a healing life—thread by thread, moment by moment—a tapestry stitched from courage, intuition, and curiosity. Let this be the start of your reclamation. A return. A remembering of what your body has been aching to say and what your spirit has longed to feel. And the version you are crafting? *It is entirely your own.* Sacred, beautiful, powerful, and wildly personal. A living, breathing map you are hand detailing back to yourself.

And that, well, that is no small thing, friend.

In fact, it's exactly what the world needs more of. And never forget: Just as mine has been . . . your survival/health reclamation story will one day become a lantern for someone else, flickering quietly, bravely, guiding them through the thickets you've already walked.

CHAPTER 14

# FALLING BACK IN LOVE WITH YOUR BODY

Many years ago, during what felt like a never-ending loop of flare-ups and hospitalizations (think Groundhog Day but with rashes and fevers), I found myself in a completely fractured relationship with my body. And when I say fractured, I mean full-on breakup status. I wanted no part of it: the illness or the vessel that carried it, or the future it seemed to be sabotaging. My body felt like a separate entity entirely, something I spoke about like an ex I was still mad at.

How could I possibly love something that felt like it was hurting me on purpose? And really, if I am being honest, if another person had caused the kind of hurt and frustration my body had, I would've cut ties and never looked back. A restraining order most definitely would have been filed.

If you've lived in a body wracked with pain, exhaustion, and all manner of frustrating symptoms for months, years, or even decades, you understand these feelings intimately. It starts to feel like your body seriously dislikes you, or at the very least, is engaged in some passive-aggressive grudge match. But here's the radical truth your inner narrative might not have whispered yet: *Your body doesn't hate you.* It never has. In fact, it's been fighting for you this whole time. It may be confused, overwhelmed, or downright dramatic, but it's not malicious.

And part of why we internalize this "my body is the enemy" narrative is due to how chronic illness is framed in medical language and culture. Phrases like "your body is attacking itself" or "your body has just gone rogue" are tossed around so casually they might as well be printed on a coffee mug. And sure, maybe sometimes they are said without much thought, believing these phrases are more shorthand explanations of complex disease responses, but these negative statements become the root of an eventual emotional rupture.

Because the idea that your own body is sabotaging you plants deep seeds of fear, mistrust, and grief.

If every symptom is interpreted as an attack, if every flare is framed as betrayal, is it any wonder you start to believe your body is out to get you? Sadly though, this belief creates a dangerous inner ecosystem, one rooted in shame, self-blame, and constant hypervigilance. And here's the kicker: that state of fight-or-flight you stay in while mentally battling your body? It increases inflammation. It spikes cortisol. It makes many symptoms greater in severity.

But what if we rewrote the story?

Because our body isn't the enemy here. Our illness is. And what if we stopped and drew a line in the sand today and decided to reframe these harmful statements? What if we decided to say instead . . . our body is confused? That our body's security system's alarms are going off at the wrong times?

What if, instead of seeing your immune system as an internal terrorist, you saw it as an overzealous guard dog? This is the analogy I used in my TEDx talk on chronic illness because it paints such a clear picture for people who are healthy.[1] What if that enthusiastic dog loves you so fiercely it's accidentally attacking its *own house* to keep you safe. The poor beast missed the memo and is now chewing on the curtains and the couch, and going after Grandma, thinking it's actually protecting you from intruders, that it's actually keeping you safe.

The intention is there, it's just . . . *a bit misdirected.*

Once I let this reframe settle in my mind, I began to notice how brutally I spoke to myself and my body on a regular basis. So, I started tracking my thoughts for a week—just one week—and I was horrified at myself. There I was, just jotting down every time I had a negative comment about my health, body, or symptoms. Spoiler alert: *It was a lot.* And it was a lot based on the ones I caught myself thinking! The sheer volume of self-criticism was staggering, and the worst part was that I hadn't even noticed doing this to myself before this moment. I had been sick for so long and angry at my body for decades, that it had become everyday background noise.

And I stood there in awe thinking, *Marisa, you have been verbally abusing yourself for decades.* It broke my heart.

I would *never, ever* speak to a friend the way I was speaking to myself. And yet, I hurled blame and resentment at my body like it was some unreliable roommate who kept eating my snacks, missing rent, and wrecking my plans. No wonder our relationship felt hostile.

There are mountains of research backing up how shame and negative self-talk directly affect our physical health, by the way. (You know I love a good data point; it's the journalist in me.) Science is clear that internalized stress and negative self-talk has negative effects on one's overall health, stress hormones, and inflammation levels.[2] In the same way that how we speak to plants will produce an effect on their quality of life, having a constant inner dialogue of "I hate my body" or "My body will never function normally" can make you feel physically worse and we all know we don't need to feel worse.

Amazingly, the opposite is true. Research suggests that positive emotions and embracing a sense of wellbeing correlate to lower levels of inflammation, with that study highlighting that people who find small positive moments each day have lower levels of inflammatory markers and stress hormones in their blood.[3]

Furthermore, one neuroscientific review on self-compassion shared that when we stop mentally attacking ourselves, we can down-regulate our fight or flight response and get out of hypervigilance mode.[4] Simply put: Being kinder to yourself, finding small moments of joy, and speaking lovingly to yourself can translate to physically and mentally feeling better. Your body literally responds to the spirit in which you treat it.

Let that sink in: Speaking to yourself kindly is *healing*.

So, how do we start repairing this fractured relationship?

One of the first shifts I made was changing how I interpreted the symptoms I was feeling. Instead of seeing them as continuous acts of betrayal, I started seeing them as messages. Little love notes from my body saying, "Hey, something's off. I really need a bit of support here."

Instead of saying, "Ugh, my joints are flaring again. My body is just broken," I began saying, "My body is inflamed today. I wonder what it's reacting to." Instead of complaining, "My body is acting crazy again, now with a horrible migraine!" I started saying, "I think my body is letting me know it's overwhelmed right now; maybe I need to turn off the lights and rest for a bit." And no, that shift in words didn't make the pain magically disappear. But it did soften the tone between me and my body. It turned an accusation into a conversation. It helped me step out of creating an atmosphere of self-blame, shame, and mistrust. Because healing won't be happening in an atmosphere filled with any of that.

The more I practiced these reframes, these healthier responses, the more I noticed something beautiful: The anger started to loosen its grip. The bitterness eased up. I began to feel less like a victim of my body and more like a teammate.

This reframe isn't fluff. It's brain retraining. It's neuroplasticity in action. And every time you choose to say something kind to your body, even if it's small, even if it feels silly or awkward, you're reinforcing a new pathway of trust and care.

Need a few phrases to start with? Try something like this—in your own authentic and unique voice, of course:

- "I am not fighting my body; my body and I are fighting this illness together."
- "I am grateful for the ways my body showed up for me today."
- "I believe my body is doing its best trying to keep me safe, even if it gets confused at times."
- "My symptoms are signals from my body, not betrayals. I choose to listen and respond to them with care."
- "I am grateful for every day my body carries me and choose to love my body as it battles pain and fatigue."

When symptoms arise, you can even try a quick exercise where you place your hand on your chest or gently over the area that's hurting. Say, "I hear you, body. I'm listening. What do you need from me right now?" Yes, it might feel weird at first. You might giggle or roll your eyes. That's okay. Humor and awkwardness are allowed here. Healing doesn't have to be solemn.

Because analogies are my love language, I want you to picture this: Your body is like a tired best friend who has carried you through every single day of your life. It breathed for you, walked you into every room, fought off every infection, kept your heart beating. And sometimes, yes, it gets things wrong (don't we all occasionally get things wrong?) but it has never stopped showing up. Would you berate that best friend for struggling? Or would you hold their hand, wipe their tears, and say, "You've done so much. Thank you. I'm here now. Let's get through this together."

And yet, when it comes to ourselves, especially with invisible and chronic illnesses, we are so quick to turn harsh. So quick to blame. The shame spiral is real and it's not just painful; it's toxic and it stalls the healing process.

So, let's call it out and break the cycle. Because, and I need you to hear this: You did not cause this illness. You didn't bring your illness on by thinking the wrong thoughts or eating the wrong food or being too stressed. You didn't manifest it with bad vibes. No matter what society, or that one clueless and unempathetic relative has to say, if you take one thing away from this chapter, from this book, let it be this: **This. Is. Not. Your. Fault.** Period. Full stop.

Our culture loves tidy cause-and-effect narratives. It helps people feel safe, as if they can avoid illness by making the "right" choices. People are so uncomfortable when talking about illness or mortality in our society, they often put blame on the person who is ill; "They eat poorly so they got diabetes," or "They never sleep so their heart gave out." Then, those of us who are in fact ill, absorb this blame and it often goes inward, causing more emotional distress and no surprise . . . more symptoms!

It's a cruel irony that can often occur with chronic illness: You are already suffering from a painful and life-changing chronic disease and then on top of that, you begin carrying shame thinking you somehow caused it. And this shame has very real effects on the physical being. In fact, research confirms that feelings of shame and self-blame when it comes to a diagnosis are often associated with higher levels of anxiety, distress, and depression.[5] It's clear to see, nothing good comes from this shame spiraling thought cycle, and it just piles more guilt onto a body and mind that is already under so much pressure and pain.

This bizarre logic that it's the patient that is to blame for the diagnosis fails the moment we zoom out. Healthy people get sick all the time. Children get cancer. Athletes are diagnosed with autoimmune diseases. Strong and seemingly healthy people in the prime of their lives suddenly die. Life is unpredictable, and illness doesn't check if you've been "good."

The bottom line is this: You are not being punished and you are not broken. You are a whole, brave, breathtakingly resilient human living in a body that's doing the best it can.

So, what now? How do we move from living in patterns of shame and anger toward our body to a new season of forgiveness and full-on love? And let's clarify really quickly: Forgiveness doesn't mean you're okay with being sick. Not at all! You can hate the illness and what it does *and* still choose not to hate yourself or your body.

Forgiving your body isn't saying "yay, illness!"; it's saying, "I refuse to keep poisoning my own well with bitterness." You're acknowledging that holding yourself responsible was unfair and harmful, so you're laying that burden down. Fully. You can still pursue treatments, fight for wellness, and even feel angry about the situation at times, but you direct that anger at the right target (the disease, the circumstances), never at yourself, and never at your body.

To help us move forward with greater love toward our body, we can write a letter. A love letter, to be exact.

I know you are likely rolling some serious eyes at me right now, but I'm being serious. A beautifully honest, tender, messy, emotional letter to your body. Because you deserve to hear those words, *from yourself.*

Think of this letter as a truce. A peace treaty. A declaration of commitment to start showing up for your body differently.

As we move into the final act of this book, writing a love letter to your body, carry this knowledge with you: You've come so far in challenging deep-seated beliefs. It's heavy work, untangling shame and blame. Give yourself credit for even *reading* this, because it means you're willing to heal not just physically, but emotionally. That is brave and beautiful.

## An Act of Love: Writing a Love Letter to Your Body

It's totally normal to feel awkward or even sad about this exercise. But I promise you with every fiber of my being, it will be incredibly cathartic. There's something almost magical about writing; the act of putting feelings into words can transform those feelings. Research has shown that writing about our emotions and experiences helps us process them and can even improve our physical health. Students who wrote about their traumas for just a few days had fewer doctor visits and needed less pain medication in the months that followed.[6] And, research in expressive writing has found this exercise to reduce stress and *strengthen the immune system.*[7] Think of this love letter assignment as giving your heart, mind, *and* body a bit of healing.

You may be asking right now: why a letter, and why full of love? Well, a letter is personal, intimate, and directed at someone, in this specific case, your body. It's not a journal entry or a generic affirmation; it's communication. And making it loving is key because, after months, years or even decades of chronic illness, chances are your relationship with your body could use some TLC.

See, your body hears your self-talk through complex brain-body feedback loops. But many of us talk to our bodies only to curse them ("Ugh, why won't you just function?!") or to command them ("Get up, we have to go to work; I don't care if you're tired"). But how often do we stop to *thank* our bodies, or say "I love you"? So think of this love letter as an offering of peace and appreciation to the vessel that has carried you thus far.

### *Penning Your Love Letter*

First, there is no wrong way to write this letter. It's for your eyes and your ears only. But here's a simple guide to help you get started if you feel stuck:

- **Set the Scene:** Find a quiet, comfortable space. Maybe play soft music if that soothes you or light a candle. Have some tissues handy; it's very possible emotions might arise.
- **Acknowledge the Journey:** Start by acknowledging what you and your body have been through together. This could be something like: "These past few years have been incredibly rough, haven't they?" or "I know I haven't always been compassionate to you, and you've been in pain." Recognize and state the struggles openly, there is no judgment here, just you and your truth.

- **Express Gratitude:** Thank your body for the things it *has* done and continues to do. This can be powerful because chronic illness often makes us focus on what's going wrong. Deliberately turn to what's still going right. For example: "Thank you, body, for breathing every day, continuing each heartbeat, even when it hurts and you are exhausted." Or, "Thank you to my legs for carrying me to the kitchen this morning, even though they felt like 100-pound weights." No act is too small to thank. "Thank you, immune system, because I know you're only trying to protect me, even if you get confused at times. Thank you, digestive system, for working so hard to process all of the food I eat." Find whatever you genuinely appreciate—there is always something, even if it's just "thank you for hanging on this long."
- **Validate the Pain:** A love letter doesn't mean glossing over the hard stuff. Be honest about what has hurt. "I'm sorry you've had to endure so many needles, so many medications and IV treatments, so much fatigue, or so many doctors that didn't believe you were hurting." You can even voice frustration, lovingly: "Sometimes I feel so mad at you for being sick, but I realize you're suffering too." This is the part where real talk and tears can flow. It's okay to admit "I've felt betrayed by you at times, and you have probably felt the same way." Getting these feelings out in the open, on paper, is like lancing a boil—it releases pressure. Just do it gently, with the intention of understanding, not accusing.
- **Apologize and Forgive:** If you realize you've been very harsh on your body, you might include an apology. "I'm sorry for calling you ugly names and thinking you were my enemy."

- **Make a Commitment to Friendship:** Now it's time to shift to a truly hopeful tone. Write about how you want your relationship to be going forward. Maybe: "I promise to listen to you better from now on and acknowledge the signals you send to me through symptoms or fatigue." Or, "I want us to work as a team, not fight each other." You might commit to treating your body with more respect. Think of these commitments as re-establishing trust.
- **Show Love and Appreciation:** End the letter with words of love or at least acceptance. If "I love you" to your body feels like too much right now, that's okay . . . maybe "I appreciate you" or "I am learning to love you" or "I see how strong you are, and I respect you" is more fitting at this moment. A year from now you may want to write another letter and you may have a completely different relationship with your body by then.

Remember, this letter is *for you*. You don't have to show it to a soul though you might choose to share it with a therapist or a close friend at some point. The act of writing it is what matters.

To inspire you to move forward with this exercise, I am letting you into a private piece of my world. A love letter I have penned to my own body:

> To the strongest little body I know,
>
> I don't even know where to begin. Honestly, since birth, we've been through hell, you and me. And because it's been ongoing for so many years, I became stuck in a pattern of anger and mistrust toward you. I realize I haven't given you enough credit. Any credit, to be exact. And because of this, I

need to tell you something: I am so very sorry. For decades, I have treated you like the enemy. I have cursed you, disowned you, distanced myself from you like you were a stranger I was forced to carry around. Still, you breathed. Still, you beat your heart. Still, you tried. You kept trying for me. I blamed you for these illnesses I've been diagnosed with, when deep down, you have been suffering terribly right alongside of me.

I've called you broken. Weak. Failing. I told people, "My body is an absolute disaster," like I wasn't talking about a living thing that has carried me every single day of my life. I told myself you betrayed me, but that was a lie I needed to believe. It felt easier than sitting with the grief of what was lost. What we used to be. What we couldn't get back.

I miss our younger days. I miss how we biked for hours, swam endlessly in the warm ocean, laughed without checking in with symptoms first. We weren't well even then, but we didn't know the worst of it yet. We had stolen freedoms: beach days and long walks, juice boxes and TV dinners that didn't knock us over with a plethora of symptoms afterward. I took those days for granted. I didn't know they were numbered.

Now, on days when I can't stand without holding onto the wall, or when the shower leaves our muscles trembling and breath short, I marvel that you still carry me. You still show up, even when I don't want to.

So this letter is both an apology and a thank you.

Thank you, feet and legs, for moving even when you feel like concrete, when there is so much pain, I can't fathom how you take one more step. Thank you, lungs, for giving me breath even when air feels like a luxury—despite asthma, despite lupus, despite the paralyzed vocal cord. You've fought for every inhale. Overworked and struggling during many moments, you still provide air and life for me all day long. Thank you, immune system, weird as it sounds, for being on the constant lookout for any germs—you *over*-pounce sometimes, and it causes me pain, but I understand it's because you're vigilant. You think you're protecting me from threats and you want to keep me safe. I appreciate the sentiment, even though I also want to say if you want to relax a bit and just chill a little more, I'd really like that!

Up until the last few years, I can honestly say I've worked against you many times. I pulled away in pain and rage, screamed at you in the dark, spoke to you in a way I wouldn't dare speak to someone I love. But it wasn't really hatred; it was all fear. I was scared, and anger felt so much easier. Easier than admitting I didn't know what was happening to us. Easier than facing the truth: I love being alive, and I'm terrified of losing my life. I think maybe you've been scared too. Scanning for danger in every corner, sounding the alarms even when the coast is clear.

We've both been trying to survive the best way we know how.

And so, I want to ask for your forgiveness. Forgive me for turning my back on you. For punishing you with overwork, silence, rage at times. For the names I called you in the dark, while we stared at hospital walls. For the nights I begged you to shut down and just give up already, because I didn't know how much longer I could carry the weight of it all.

You are not the villain here. You never were.

Forgive me for calling you "broken" and "a hot mess" and "a disaster"—You are none of these. You are doing the best you can under absolutely insane circumstances. You are fighting a war nobody else can see, and you keep going day after day, almost fifty years now. I told the world you were a liability, but the truth is, you're a living miracle. After decade after decade of suffering, you're still standing. That makes you one badass warrior.

Moving forward, I am not fighting you anymore. From now on, I am *with you.*

I promise to listen when you signal in whispers, so you don't have to scream. I promise to stop pushing past your breaking point just to prove I'm still functional. I will rest without guilt. I will nourish us well. I will not ignore your cries anymore.

You have never once stopped trying to keep me alive.

So, I will never again stop trying to love you.

It won't be perfect. There will be days I fail at this. But I'll always return to this promise.

Thank you for not giving up on me.

Thank you for surviving every time I thought we wouldn't.

Thank you for the memories I got to make in this life because you endured and carried me.

Thank you for being my home, even when I treated you like a prison.

You are a beautiful vessel that has offered me the opportunity of enjoying such a blessed life, despite our hardships. I love you, body. Not because you're perfect. I love you because you never quit. I love you because you are astonishing.

I love you because you are mine,

We're going to figure this out—together; one breath, one heartbeat, one day at a time.

Marisa

In this moment, take a deep breath. What thoughts or emotions stirred up when you read my letter? Maybe your eyes welled up; maybe you thought "Marisa is a bit bonkers" . . . or maybe both. There's no "right" reaction. Writing a letter like this brings up a lot of emotions: grief for what's been lost, relief from unspoken feelings finally voiced, hope for a more loving future. All of it is valid.

If you need a break before writing yours, that's okay. But do come back to it when you're ready, even if it's just jotting a few bullet-point notes to your body to start. You might be surprised by the outcome. Many people find that after writing such a letter, they feel a softening towards themselves.

## Embracing Your Journey Forward

As we close this chapter, and this book, I want you to take a moment to appreciate how far you've come. Not just in reading these pages, but in your life with chronic illness. You have survived every single day up to now. *You have survived.* The strength required to live in an uncooperative body is tremendous. The fact that you are still seeking ways to love yourself in the midst of all this means you are incredibly resilient.

Keep that love letter somewhere safe. You might even choose to reread it on days when you feel especially disconnected or challenging symptoms have you beginning to spiral. It can be a beautiful reminder of the truce and friendship you are forging with your body. Some days you won't feel the love, and that is okay. You don't have to maintain constant positivity. Self-love is not a destination; it's a practice. You're going to have ups and downs. On the hard days, try not to default back to self-blame. Maybe all you'll manage is, "Today I hate that these symptoms are present, but tomorrow is a new day and I am going to give my body rest." That loving reframe is in itself an act of compassion.

As a community (and yes, you have a community; so many of us out here are walking parallel paths, even if we've never met), we stand in solidarity with you. When I say you're not alone, I mean it. There are countless hearts out here that understand what you're going through right at this very moment.

Think of this book as one friend extending a hand to you; there are others. We're all learning to be a little kinder to ourselves, learning to see our bodies not as the enemy but as a wounded friend that needs our comfort.

So, if you ever doubt it, come back to these words. Hear this voice (my voice, but also the collective voice of chronic illness warriors everywhere) saying: "You are not to blame. Your body loves you and is doing its best. You deserve gentleness, especially from yourself." On days when you can't believe that, let us hold that truth for you until you can. And on days when you *can* believe it, soak it in fully. Share it with someone else who is hurting.

And dear reader, there is something I have to say that I want you to grab onto and never let go off, even in the darkest moments: You are so worthy of love—unwavering, unconditional love—regardless of illness or ability. Chronic illness may have changed your life, but it will never, ever change your *worth*.

To walk this road beside you has been one of the greatest honors of my life. In a world that rarely understands us, we have found each other—and that is no small miracle. The chronic illness community is stitched together with invisible thread: resilience, humor, grief, grit, and the kind of compassion that can only be born from shared suffering.

This community has carried me, and I hope, in these pages, I've carried you too. As you rise, even slowly, even shakily, don't forget the ones still curled up at the beginning of their story. Reach back. Offer a hand, a word, a knowing nod. This is how we heal—together, endlessly passing the light forward in the dark.

XOXO<br>
Your forever spoonie bestie,<br>
Marisa

# ACKNOWLEDGMENTS

This book began long before words ever hit the page—back in those quiet, confusing moments when illness first made its unwelcome entrance into my life. I didn't know then that the pain, the questions, and the slow resilience I was building would one day shape something that could help others navigate their own health journey. But . . . here we are. And if you're holding this book in your hands, that means healing in your life—in some form, at some stage—is already beginning. That alone makes me emotional.

I am only able to do the work I love—write, speak, advocate, create—because I am held up by grace. First, to God, who continues to carry me and remind me that my voice still matters, even on the hardest days. To my beautiful chronic illness community: thank you for letting me walk alongside you. You are fierce and soft and everything in between, and it is an honor to be in this with you.

To my family, who has loved me through every detour and diagnosis, and to my husband, whose steady presence and unique views on life keep me grounded when everything in my atmosphere feels upside down. To my TEDx family—you changed my life. And to the strong, spicy, laugh-till-we-snort friends who root for me even when I ghost them during a flare: thank you for staying. Thank you for loving me and being my forever cheerleading squad. And to my favorite cousin, Frankie, there's no one I'd rather be experiencing this wild ride of life with!

This book would still be a Word doc in the abyss of my very cluttered desktop if not for the incredible humans who believed in me and this message. Laura Strachan, thank you for being my literary lighthouse and agent, and to Daniela Rapp and Tony Lyons at Skyhorse—your belief in this work, and in the power of hope for those with chronic illness, means the world to me.

To every single one of you who said "keep going" when I felt like throwing in the towel: thank you. Your encouragement helped this book come alive. And now, my hope is it goes out into the world and helps someone else do the same.

# RESOURCES

## Resources for Navigating Chronic Illness

### *Medical-Grade Supplement Brands*

- Metagenics—www.metagenics.com
- Thorne—www.thorne.com
- Standard Process—www.standardprocess.com
- Pure Encapsulations—www.pureencapsulations.com
- Designs for Health—www.designsforhealth.com
- Integrative Therapeutics—www.integrativepro.com

## Career and Disability Support

- Social Security Disability Benefits (SSA)—www.ssa.gov/benefits/disability
- Job Accommodation Network (JAN)—askjan.org
- abilityJOBS—www.abilityjobs.com
- Ticket to Work (SSA)—choosework.ssa.gov

## Functional Medicine and Nutrition Providers

- Institute for Functional Medicine (IFM)—www.ifm.org/find-a-practitioner

- Academy of Integrative Health & Medicine—members.aihm.org/find-a-provider
- Academy of Nutrition and Dietetics—www.eatright.org/find-a-nutrition-expert
- Institute for Natural Medicine—www.findanaturaldoctor.com

## Healthy Food Suppliers (Chronic Illness Friendly)

- Thrive Market—www.thrivemarket.com
- Vitacost—www.vitacost.com
- iHerb—www.iherb.com
- Azure Standard—www.azurestandard.com
- Misfits Market—www.misfitsmarket.com
- US Wellness Meats—www.grasslandbeef.com

## Free or Low-Cost Online Learning and Skill Building

- Coursera—www.coursera.org
- edX—www.edx.org
- Khan Academy—www.khanacademy.org
- MIT OpenCourseWare (OCW)—ocw.mit.edu
- OpenLearn (Open University)—www.open.edu/openlearn
- Alison—www.alison.com

## Additional Supportive Resources

- The Mighty—www.themighty.com
- Health Union—www.health-union.com
- Folia Health—www.foliahealth.com
- Inspire—www.inspire.com
- PatientsLikeMe—www.patientslikeme.com
- Invisible Disabilities Association—www.invisibledisabilities.org

- Chronic Disease Coalition—www.chronicdiseasecoalition.org
- Center for Chronic Illness—www.thecenterforchronicillness.org

## Companies that Pay Patients for Health Insights and Experiences

- TheInsighters—www.theinsighters.com
- Folia Health—www.foliahealth.com
- JoinedBio—www.Joined.bio
- Rare Patient Voice—www.rarepatientvoice.com

# REFERENCES


**Chapter Two**

1 Autoimmune Association. (2021). "Path to a Rare Disease Diagnoses." The Autoimmune Association. https://autoimmune.org/resource-center/autoimmune-summit/2021-autoimmune-summit/path-to-rare-disease-diagnoses/.

2 Smith, C. D., & Cyr, M. (1988). "The History of Lupus Erythematosus: From Hippocrates to Osler." *Rheumatic Disease Clinics of North America*, 14, 1–14. https://scispace.com/papers/the-history-of-lupus-erythematosus-from-hippocrates-to-osler-4mx39sbim4.

3 *The Holy Bible*, Contemporary English Version (CEV). (n.d.). Matthew 6:34. Bible Gateway. https://www.biblegateway.com/passage/?search=Matthew%206%3A34&version=CEV.

**Chapter Three**

1 Josell, R. (2025, April 22). "What Are the Stages of Grief?" *Cleveland Clinic*. https://health.clevelandclinic.org/5-stages-of-grief.

**Chapter Four**

1 Colangelo, K., Haig, S., Bonner, A., Zelenietz, C., & Pope, J. (2011). "Self-Reported Flaring Varies during the Menstrual Cycle in Systemic Lupus Erythematosus Compared with Rheumatoid Arthritis and Fibromyalgia." *Rheumatology (Oxford)*, *50*(4), 703–708. https://pubmed.ncbi.nlm.nih.gov/21115463/.

2 He, J., Guo, Y., Chen, J., Xu, J., & Zhu, X. (2025). "Exploring the Correlation between UVB Sensitivity and SLE Activity: Insights into UVB-driven Pathogenesis in Lupus Erythematosus." *Journal of Autoimmunity, 153*, 103393. https://www.sciencedirect.com/science/article/abs/pii/S0896841125000381.

3 Watanabe, Y., & Yamaguchi, Y. (2022). "Drug Allergy and Autoimmune Diseases." *Allergology International, 71*(2), 179–184. https://www.sciencedirect.com/science/article/pii/S1323893022000065?via%3Dihub.

4 Krishna, M. T., Subramanian, A., Adderley, N. J., Zemedikun, D. T., Gkoutos, G. V., & Nirantharakumar, K. (2019). "Allergic Diseases and Long-term Risk of Autoimmune Disorders: Longitudinal Cohort Study and Cluster Analysis." *European Respiratory Journal, 54*(5), 1900476. https://pubmed.ncbi.nlm.nih.gov/31413164/.

5 D'Auria, E., Minutoli, M., Colombo, A., Sartorio, M. U. A., Zunica, F., Zuccotti, G., & Lougaris, V. (2023). "Allergy and Autoimmunity in Children: Non-mutually Exclusive Diseases—A narrative review." *Frontiers in Pediatrics, 11*, Article 1239365. https://www.frontiersin.org/journals/pediatrics/articles/10.3389/fped.2023.1239365/full.

**Chapter Six**

1 DePaulo, B. (2025, March 9). "Why More Marriages End when Wives Become Ill than When Husbands Do." *Psychology Today.* https://www.psychologytoday.com/us/blog/living-single/202503/why-more-marriages-end-when-wives-become-ill-than-when-husbands-do.

2 National Academies of Sciences, Engineering, and Medicine. (2024). *Advancing Research on Chronic Conditions in Women*. National Academies Press. https://www.ncbi.nlm.nih.gov/books/NBK604853/.

3 Cunningham, S. J., & Patel, S. S. (2003, January 15). "Chronic Illness and Sexual Functioning." *American Family Physician, 67*(2), 347–354. https://www.aafp.org/pubs/afp/issues/2003/0115/p347.html.

4 Maturitas. (2022). "Patients with Chronic Diseases: Is Sexual Health Brought up by General Practitioners during Appointments?" *Maturitas, 165*, 24-30. https://www.sciencedirect.com/science/article/pii/S0378512222000275.

**Chapter Seven**

1 National Center on Health, Physical Activity and Disability. (2025). "Spoon Theory: A New Way to Think about Your Daily Energy." https://www.nchpad.org/resources/spoon-theory-a-new-way-to-think-about-your-daily-energy/.

2 Little, B. (2020, July 24). "When the 'Capitol Crawl' Dramatized the Need for Americans with Disabilities Act." *History.* A&E Television Networks. https://www.history.com/articles/americans-with-disabilities-act-1990-capitol-crawl.

3 Job Accommodation Network. (n.d.). "Disability Disclosure." U.S. Department of Labor, Office of Disability Employment Policy. https://askjan.org/topics/Disability-Disclosure.cfm.

4 WebMD. (n.d.). "Lupus Photosensitivity and UV Light." WebMD. https://www.webmd.com/lupus/lupus-photosensitivity-uv.

5 Social Security Administration. (2021). "Outcomes of Applications for Disability Benefits." In *Annual Statistical Report on the Social Security Disability Insurance Program, 2020.* https://www.ssa.gov/policy/docs/statcomps/di_asr/2020/sect04.html.


## Chapter Eight


1 Nutt, D. J., & Malizia, A. L. (2004). "Structural and Functional Brain Changes in Posttraumatic Stress Disorder." *The Journal of Clinical Psychiatry, 65* (Suppl. 1), 11–17. https://pubmed.ncbi.nlm.nih.gov/14728092/.

2 Johns Hopkins Medicine. (2025, March 10). "Worldwide Study Finds High Rates of Depression and Anxiety in People with Chronic Pain." https://www.hopkinsmedicine.org/news/newsroom/news-releases/2025/03/worldwide-study-finds-high-rates-of-depression-and-anxiety-in-people-with-chronic-pain.


## Chapter Ten


1 Ramirez, G. A., Cardamone, C., Lettieri, S., Fredi, M., & Mormile, I. (2025). "Clinical and Pathophysiological Tangles Between Allergy and Autoimmunity: Deconstructing an Old Dichotomic Paradigm." *Clinical Reviews in Allergy & Immunology, 68*(1), 13 https://pmc.ncbi.nlm.nih.gov/articles/PMC11814061/.

2 Ng, A. E., & Boersma, P. (2023). "Diagnosed Allergic Conditions in Adults: United States, 2021" (NCHS Data Brief No. 460). National Center for Health Statistics. https://www.cdc.gov/nchs/products/databriefs/db460.htm.

3 ThermoFisherScientific. (n.d.). "CanAllergiesChangeoverTime?" AllergyInsider. https://www.thermofisher.com/allergy/wo/en/living-with-allergies/understanding-allergies/can-allergies-change-over-time.html.

4 Cleveland Clinic. (2024). "Glutamine." https://my.clevelandclinic.org/health/articles/glutamine.

5 Stamets, P., & Zwickey, H. (2014). "Medicinal Mushrooms: Ancient Remedies Meet Modern Science." *Integrative Medicine: A Clinician's Journal, 13*(1), 46–47. https://pmc.ncbi.nlm.nih.gov/articles/PMC4684114/.

6 Jayachandran, M., Xiao, J., & Xu, B. (2017). "A Critical Review on Health Promoting Benefits of Edible Mushrooms through Gut Microbiota." *International Journal of Molecular Sciences, 18*(9), 1934. https://pmc.ncbi.nlm.nih.gov/articles/PMC5618583/.

7 University of Washington School of Medicine. (2022, July 6). "Butyrate in Microbiome Abates a Host of Ills, Studies Find." UW Medicine Newsroom. https://newsroom.uw.edu/blog/butyrate-microbiome-abates-host-ills-studies-find#.

8 Singh, V., Lee, G., Son, H., Koh, H., Kim, E. S., Unno, T., & Shin, J.-H. (2023). "Butyrate Producers, 'The Sentinel of Gut': Their Intestinal Significance with and beyond Butyrate, and Prospective Use as Microbial Therapeutics." Frontiers in Microbiology, 13, Article 1103836. https://pmc.ncbi.nlm.nih.gov/articles/PMC9877435/.

9 Sroka, N., Rydzewska-Rosołowska, A., Kakareko, K., Rosołowski, M., Głowińska, I., & Hryszko, T. (2022). "Show Me What You Have Inside—the Complex Interplay between SIBO and Multiple Medical Conditions—a Systematic Review." *Nutrients*, 15(1), Article 90. https://pmc.ncbi.nlm.nih.gov/articles/PMC9824151/.

**Chapter Eleven**

1 Bhusal, K. K., Magar, S. K., Thapa, R., Lamsal, A., Bhandari, S., Maharjan, R., Shrestha, S., & Shrestha, J. (2022). "Nutritional and Pharmacological Importance of Stinging Nettle (*Urtica dioica* L.): A Review." *Heliyon, 8*(6), e09717. https://pmc.ncbi.nlm.nih.gov/articles/PMC9253158/.

2 Cohen, M. M. (2014). "Tulsi—*Ocimum Sanctum*: A Herb for All Reasons." *Journal of Ayurveda and Integrative Medicine, 5*(4), 251–259. https://pmc.ncbi.nlm.nih.gov/articles/PMC4296439/.

3 Jamshidi, N., & Cohen, M. M. (2017). "The Clinical Efficacy and Safety of Tulsi in Humans: A Systematic Review of the Literature." *Evidence-Based Complementary and Alternative Medicine, 2017*, Article 9217567. https://pmc.ncbi.nlm.nih.gov/articles/PMC5376420/.

4 National Center for Complementary and Integrative Health. (2025). "Astragalus: Usefulness and Safety." U.S. Department of Health and Human Services. https://www.nccih.nih.gov/health/astragalus.

5 Meixner, M. (2025, September 2). "Astragalus: An Ancient Root with Health Benefits." Healthline. https://www.healthline.com/nutrition/astragalus.

6 AlDehlawi, H., & Jazzar, A. (2023). "The Power of Licorice (*Radix glycyrrhizae*) to Improve Oral Health: A Comprehensive Review of Its Pharmacological Properties and Clinical Implications." *Healthcare, 11*(21), 2887. https://pmc.ncbi.nlm.nih.gov/articles/PMC10648065/.

7 Arshad, M. T., Maqsood, S., Ikram, A., & Abdullahi, M. A. (2025). "Functional, Nutraceutical, and Health-Endorsing Perspectives of Ashwagandha." *eFood, 6*(3), Article e70061. https://iadns.onlinelibrary.wiley.com/doi/10.1002/efd2.70061.

8 Wiciński, M., Fajkiel-Madajczyk, A., Kurant, Z., Kurant, D., Gryczka, K., Falkowski, M., & *et al.* (2023). "Can Ashwagandha Benefit the Endocrine System?—A Review." *International Journal of Molecular Sciences, 24*(22), 16513. https://pmc.ncbi.nlm.nih.gov/articles/PMC10671406/.

9 Kraft, S., Buchenauer, L., Polte, T., & Peters, A. (2021). "Mold, Mycotoxins and a Dysregulated Immune System: A Combination of Concern?" *International Journal of Molecular Sciences, 22*(22), 12269. https://pmc.ncbi.nlm.nih.gov/articles/PMC8619365/.

10 Environmental Working Group. (2008, September 24). "Teen Girls' Body Burden of Hormone-Altering Cosmetics Chemicals." https://www.ewg.org/research/teen-girls-body-burden-hormone-altering-cosmetics-chemicals.

11 Environmental Working Group. (2023, July 25). "What Is Fragrance?" https://www.ewg.org/news-insights/news/2023/07/what-fragrance.

12 Foley, J. (2024, June 25). "What Are 'Natural Flavors,' and Are They Really Natural?" GoodRx. https://www.goodrx.com/well-being/diet-nutrition/what-are-natural-flavors.

13 Cleveland Clinic. (2023). "Lymphatic system: Function, Conditions & Disorders." https://my.clevelandclinic.org/health/body/21199-lymphatic-system.

14 Shively, M. (2023, October 13). "How to Give Yourself a Lymphatic Drainage Massage." Verywell Health. https://www.verywellhealth.com/lymphatic-drainage-massage-7972279.

15 Al Jaouni, S. K., El-Fiky, E. A., Mourad, S. A., Ibrahim, N. K., Kaki, A. M., Rohaiem, S. M., Qari, M. H., Tabsh, L. M., & Aljawhari, A. A. (2017). "The Effect of Wet Cupping on Quality of Life of Adult Patients with Chronic Medical Conditions in King Abdulaziz University Hospital." *Saudi Medical Journal, 38*(1), 53–62. https://pmc.ncbi.nlm.nih.gov/articles/PMC5278066/.

16 Al Jaouni, S. K., Rohaiem, S. M., Almuhayawi, M. S., Godugu, K., Almughales, J., Kholi, S. M., Al-Raddadi, R., Bukhari, M., & Mousa, S. A. (2023). "Wet Cupping Therapy in the Modulation of Inflammation in Patients with Pain." *RPS Pharmacy and Pharmacology Reports, 2*(2), rqad004. https://academic.oup.com/rpsppr/article/2/2/rqad004/7045985.

**Chapter Twelve**

1 Shane-McWhorter, L. (2025). "Intravenous Vitamin Therapy (Myers' cocktail)." In *Merck Manuals Consumer Version*. Merck & Co., Inc. https://www.merckmanuals.com/home/special-subjects/dietary-supplements-and-vitamins/intravenous-vitamin-therapy-myers-cocktail.

2 Wasik, A. A., & Tuuminen, T. (2021). "Salt Therapy as a Complementary Method for the Treatment of Respiratory Tract Diseases, with a Focus on Mold-Related Illness." *Alternative Therapies in Health and Medicine*, 27(Suppl. 1), 223-239. https://pubmed.ncbi.nlm.nih.gov/34726628/.

3 Sutherland, A. M., Clarke, H. A., Katz, J., & Katznelson, R. (2016). "Hyperbaric Oxygen Therapy: A New Treatment for Chronic Pain?" *Pain Practice, 16*(5), 620–628. https://pubmed.ncbi.nlm.nih.gov/25988526/.

4 Bekaryssova, D., Yessirkepov, M., & Imanbaeva, A. D. (2024). "Water-Based Interventions in Rheumatic Diseases: Mechanisms, Benefits, and Clinical Applications." *Rheumatology International, 45*(1), 8. https://pubmed.ncbi.nlm.nih.gov/39733125/.

5 Zamunér, A. R., Andrade, C. P., Arca, E. A., Avila, M. A., & et al. (2019). "Impact of Water Therapy on Pain Management in Patients with Fibromyalgia: Current Perspectives." *Journal of Pain Research, 12,* 1971–2007. https://pmc.ncbi.nlm.nih.gov/articles/PMC6613198/.

6 Ko, Y. (2016). "Sebastian Kneipp and the Natural Cure Movement of Germany: Between Naturalism and Modern Medicine." *Uisahak, 25*(3), 557–590. https://pubmed.ncbi.nlm.nih.gov/28529304/.

## Chapter Thirteen

1 Haller, H., Lauche, R., Sundberg, T., Dobos, G., & Cramer, H. (2019). "Craniosacral Therapy for Chronic Pain: A Systematic Review and Meta-analysis of Randomized Controlled Trials." *BMC Musculoskeletal Disorders*, 21, 1. https://pmc.ncbi.nlm.nih.gov/articles/PMC6937867/.

2 Field, T. (2016). "Massage therapy research review." *Complementary Therapies in Clinical Practice, 24,* 19–31. https://pmc.ncbi.nlm.nih.gov/articles/PMC5564319/.

3 Al Refaei, A. (2021). "Therapeutic Massage for Hospitalized COVID-19 Patients: Potential Mechanisms and Considerations." *International Journal of Therapeutic Massage & Bodywork*, 14(1), 49–56. https://pmc.ncbi.nlm.nih.gov/articles/PMC7892330/#b2-ijtmb-14-49.

4 Li, N., Guo, Y., Gong, Y., Zhang, Y., Fan, W., Yao, K., … Dou, B. (2021). "The Anti-inflammatory Actions and Mechanisms of Acupuncture from Acupoint to Target Organs via Neuro-immune Regulation." *Journal of Inflammation Research, 14,* 7191–7224. https://pmc.ncbi.nlm.nih.gov/articles/PMC8710088/.

5 Lu, M., Sharmin, S., Tao, Y., Xia, X., Yang, G., Cong, Y., Yang, G., Jiang, J., Xiao, Y., Peng, L., Quan, J., & Xu, B. (2024). "Effectiveness of Acupuncture in Treating Patients with Pain and Mental Health Concerns: The Results of the Alberta Complementary Health Integration Project." *Frontiers in Neurology, 15,* Article 1366685. https://pmc.ncbi.nlm.nih.gov/articles/PMC11333307/.

6 McManus, D. E. (2017). "Reiki Is Better than Placebo and Has Broad Potential as a Complementary Health Therapy." *Journal of Evidence-Based Complementary & Alternative Medicine*, 22(4), 1051–1057. https://pmc.ncbi.nlm.nih.gov/articles/PMC5871310/.

7 Estevão, A. C., & Fisher, P. L. (2022). "The Role of Yoga in Inflammatory Markers: A Mini-review." *International Journal of Therapeutic Massage & Bodywork, 14*(2), 49–57. https://pmc.ncbi.nlm.nih.gov/articles/PMC8842003/.

8 Jamieson, I. A. (2023). "Grounding (earthing) as Related to Electromagnetic Hygiene: An Integrative Review." *Biomedical Journal, 46*(1), 30–40. https://pmc.ncbi.nlm.nih.gov/articles/PMC10105031/.

9 Bosman, J. T., Bood, Z. M., Scherer-Rath, M., Dörr, H., Christophe, N., Sprangers, M. A. G., & van Laarhoven, H. W. M. (2021). "The Effects of Art Therapy on Anxiety, Depression, and Quality of Life in Adults with Cancer: A Systematic Literature Review." *Supportive Care in Cancer, 29*(5), 2289–2298. https://pmc.ncbi.nlm.nih.gov/articles/PMC7981299/.

10 Raudenská, J., Šteinerová, V., Vodičková, Š., Raudenský, M., Fulková, M., Urits, I., Viswanath, O., Varrassi, G., & Javůrková, A. (2023). "Arts Therapy and Its Implications in Chronic Pain Management: A Narrative Review." *Pain and Therapy, 12*(6), 1309–1337. https://pmc.ncbi.nlm.nih.gov/articles/PMC10616022/.

11 Fu, Y., Wu, K., Zhuang, J., Chen, Y., Jia, L., Luo, Z., & Sun, R. (2025). "Music Therapy in Modulating Immune Responses and Enhancing Cancer Treatment Outcomes." *Frontiers in Immunology, 16*, 1639047. https://pmc.ncbi.nlm.nih.gov/articles/PMC12325063/.

12 Mukherjee, O., & Mutnury, S. L. (2021). "Management of Chronic Illness through Music Therapy: A Review." *Indian Journal of Health Studies, 3*(2), 55–94. https://www.researchgate.net/publication/361209287_Management_of_Chronic_Illness_through_Music_Therapy_A_Review.

13 Black, D. S., & Slavich, G. M. (2016). "Mindfulness Meditation and the Immune System: A Systematic Review of Randomized Controlled Trials." *Annals of the New York Academy of Sciences*, 1373(1), 13–24. https://pmc.ncbi.nlm.nih.gov/articles/PMC4940234/.

14 Goldsby, T. L., Goldsby, M. E., McWalters, M., & Mills, P. J. (2017). "Effects of Singing Bowl Sound Meditation on Mood, Tension, and Well-being: An Observational Study." *Journal of Evidence-Based Complementary & Alternative Medicine,* 22(3), 401–406. https://pmc.ncbi.nlm.nih.gov/articles/PMC5871151/.

15 Jors, K., Büssing, A., Hvidt, N. C., & Baumann, K. (2015). "Personal Prayer in Patients Dealing with Chronic Illness: A Review of the Research Literature." *Evidence-Based Complementary and Alternative Medicine*, 2015, Article 927973. https://www.researchgate.net/publication/272830184_Personal_Prayer_in_Patients_Dealing_with_Chronic_Illness_A_Review_of_the_Research_Literature.

16 Ironson, G., & Ahmad, S. S. (2024). "Frequency of Private Prayer Predicts Survival over 6 years in a Nationwide U.S. Sample of Individuals with a Chronic Illness." *Journal of Religion and Health,* 63(4), 2910–2923. https://pmc.ncbi.nlm.nih.gov/articles/PMC11319365/.

17 Joseph, S. (2019). "Sound Healing Using Solfeggio Frequencies." Graduate thesis. American College of Healthcare Sciences. https://www.researchgate.net/publication/333852911_Sound_Healing_using_Solfeggio_Frequencies.

**Chapter Fourteen**

1 Zeppieri, M. (2025, April). "When Illness Is Invisible, Let Curiosity Lead" [Video]. YouTube. https://www.youtube.com/watch?v=Dw__mb9fNB8&t=10s.

2 Schneiderman, N., Ironson, G., & Siegel, S. D. (2005). "Stress and Health: Psychological, Behavioral, and Biological Determinants." *Annual Review of Clinical Psychology, 1*(1), 607–628. https://pmc.ncbi.nlm.nih.gov/articles/PMC2568977/.

3 Sin, N. L., Graham-Engeland, J. E., & Almeida, D. M. (2015). "Daily Positive Events and Inflammation: Findings from the National Study of Daily Experiences." *Brain, Behavior, and Immunity, 43*, 130–138. https://pmc.ncbi.nlm.nih.gov/articles/PMC4258510/.

4 The Minded Institute. (2025, February 4). "Yoga and neuroscience: The Power of Self-talk." https://themindedinstitute.com/yoga-and-neuroscience-the-power-of-self%E2%80%91talk/#:~:text=On%20the%20flip%20side%2C%20research,being.

5 Callebaut, L., Molyneux, P., & Alexander, T. (2017). "The Relationship between Self-blame for the Onset of a Chronic Physical Health Condition and Emotional Distress: A Systematic Literature Review." *Clinical Psychology & Psychotherapy*, 24(4), 965–986. https://pubmed.ncbi.nlm.nih.gov/27925335/.

6 Harvard Health Publishing. (2011, October 11). "Writing about Emotions May Ease Stress and Trauma." Harvard Health. https://www.health.harvard.edu/healthbeat/writing-about-emotions-may-ease-stress-and-trauma.

7 American Psychological Association. (2002, June). "Writing to Heal: How Expressing Your Emotions through Writing May Benefit Your Health." *Monitor on Psychology*. https://www.apa.org/monitor/jun02/writing.

# INDEX